THE PASSION OF
FLORENCE
NIGHTINGALE

HUGH SMALL

First published 2010

Amberley Publishing Plc
Cirencester Road, Chalford,
Stroud, Gloucestershire, GL6 8PE

www.amberleybooks.com

ISBN 978-1-4456-0064-2

Typeset in 10pt on 12pt Sabon.
Typesetting and Origination by Fonthill.
Printed in the UK.

Contents

	Acknowledgements	4
	Preface	5
1.	Ambition	7
2.	At War	21
3.	Stirring Events, Romantic Dangers	33
4.	Post-Mortem	56
5.	Conversion	73
6.	Cover-Up	85
7.	'By pestilence perished before their time'	109
8.	Reputation and Myth	137
	Appendix I Differences	154
	Appendix II Sources	156
	Index	158

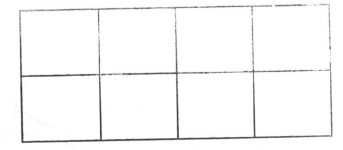

Acknowledgements

I am grateful to Radcliffes & Co., who administer the Henry Bonham Carter Will Trust, for permission to publish letters of Florence Nightingale and her family. Extracts from letters in the Greater London Record Office are printed by courtesy of the Florence Nightingale Museum Trust, London, and the Claydon Trust has allowed me to print letters from Claydon House.

Preface

Enough new material has become available in the twelve years since the publication of *Florence Nightingale, Avenging Angel* to make it necessary to revise it extensively and give it a change of direction, as expressed in the new title. The factual revelations of the 1998 publication, which were seen as astonishing at the time, are now widely accepted by scholars: that she did not discover until after the Crimean War that conditions in her hospital had contributed to the death of its patients, that the government refused to let her publish the evidence to prove it, and that she leaked the evidence to a circle of opinion-makers instead. These facts are becoming received wisdom, and the old story that she dramatically reduced the death rate at Scutari is fast being demoted to a harmless and charming legend that need not cloud the truth. This time I have been able to cut out the detailed evidence disproving what was, at the time of the previous book, a strongly held belief that she had dramatically reduced wartime mortality. There is now a more widespread awareness that Nightingale's achievements after the war, rather than those sentimentally attributed to her at Scutari, are the justification for her place in history.

So much suppressed factual material has already come to light after a century and a half that it should come as no suprise that the mutual infatuation between Nightingale and a married man during the war has been covered up until now. The affair is relevant because it helps to explain why Nightingale became blind to the real cause of the high mortality in her hospital, and why she was so deeply affected when she found out the truth. I hope that by describing some of her romantic relationships, imaginary and real, welcome and unwelcome, I can show a new and more human dimension of this remarkable Victorian.

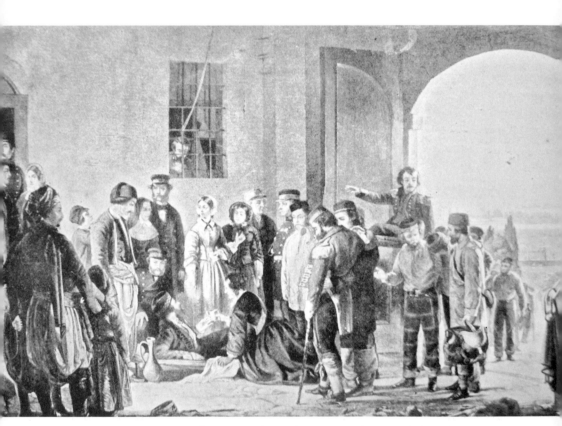

The Mission of Mercy: Florence Nightingale receiving the wounded at Scutari.
(Painting by Jerry Barrett)

CHAPTER ONE

Ambition

In her youth, Florence Nightingale dreamed of a life of heroic action, and by the strangest chance her dream was realised during the Crimean War. But unlike most women of her time who were attracted to good works, she was not satisfied with action alone. She had to step back and analyse the conduct of the war and her own role in it, with the inevitable result that she found plenty to criticise in both. Her need for both intense action and profound analysis came from the circumstances of her education and family life.

She was the younger of two sisters, born in quick succession while their wealthy parents were travelling the Continent on an extended honeymoon. Her sister was born at Naples and named Parthenope (pronounced parth-*en*-o-pee or *par*-thee for short), after a figure from Greek mythology who was said to be buried there. Florence was born one year later, in 1820, and was named after the city of her birth. Her father had been an indolent but intelligent and reflective youth who had inherited great wealth from an uncle. Her mother was a socially active beauty, who married her father for his wealth after realising that the minor aristocrat with whom she had fallen in love could not finance her extravagant lifestyle. Once the children were born, Nightingale's father spent his time avoiding his wife's attempts to integrate him into society, hiding in the Athenaeum Club in London or studying with Florence in his library. Nightingale, like her father, found society activities trivial and meaningless.

Affluent families of that time were usually highly religious and Nightingale's family had a strong Unitarian tradition. Unitarians were Christians who did not acknowledge the doctrine of the Trinity, a doctrine that was a basic test of adherence to the official established Church of England. The Unitarians' refusal to accept this creed was due to their reluctance to follow rules handed down by authority rather than a claim of superior insight into the nature of God. Another common Unitarian technique for provoking the Church of England was to deny the divinity of Christ. Until 1813, it was a criminal offence to do so in England. The Member of Parliament who persuaded the legislature to repeal this

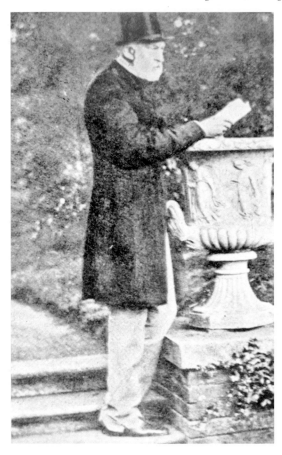

William Nightingale, Florence's father, who was seldom seen without a book, which he would read standing up.

section of the criminal law in 1813 was Florence Nightingale's maternal grandfather.

It is hard to know whether Nightingale actually considered herself a Unitarian, because members of the sect are difficult to categorise and she herself is particularly elusive. During the Crimean War she wrote to Sidney Herbert that one of the nurses had 'fallen under the Chaplain's displeasure for Socinianism – of which genus we have two'. Socinianism was the heresy committed by those Unitarians who denied the divinity of Christ. Herbert is on record as being aware that a charge of Socinianism had already been levelled at Nightingale, and so he could see that she was identifying herself as the first heretic of the pair. Perhaps she was writing playfully, but still the strength of the tradition in both her mother's and her father's family must have influenced her, and some of her medical attitudes are easier to understand when their Unitarian overtones are taken into account. The Unitarian religion is described as based on 'deeds not creeds'. Unitarians were fond of pointing out that the Trinity and other creeds did not come from the bible but were invented by earthly rulers who wanted to suppress independent thought. Nightingale herself claimed to be unqualified to guess at such details as whether God was one being or three, details which she called His *essence*. She could, she said, deduce what kind of *character* He had from the way He had created the world, and that was enough for her to be able to do His work. This is a Unitarian position. To our more cynical ears it may sound as though Unitarianism was a cunning camouflage for atheism, but Nightingale's most private writings show that she revered Christ even if she did not think him divine.

Nightingale's independence of thought made her relationship with her mother and sister difficult. She was most attached to her father who devoted much of his wealth to intellectual pursuits for himself and his daughters. Nightingale was very close to him when young, much closer than her older sister Parthenope had been. Their father had educated both of them at home, and Florence had been the better pupil. But as Nightingale grew up under his wing and began to yearn for a life of useful activity, she came to look on her father with a mixture of pity and contempt. One of her autobiographical notes written while she was still living at home reads: 'My father is a man who has never known what struggle is. Good impulses from his childhood up, having never by circumstances been forced to look into a thing, to carry it out. He has not enough to fill his faculties. When I see him eating his breakfast as if the destinies of a nation depended upon his getting done, carrying his plate about the room, delighting in being in a hurry, I say to myself how happy that man would be with a factory under his superintendence – with the interests of two or three hundred men to look after.'

She was not doing justice to her father when she said he had never 'carried anything out'. One – perhaps the only – important achievement of his life was too close for her to see. This was the education of Florence, an ambitious project that he completed at home, with the help of external tutors, and on educational trips abroad to France, Italy, and Switzerland. He accomplished far more than was necessary or considered desirable for a lady, training her in French, German, Italian, Latin, Greek, History, and Philosophy. Her father might, in different circumstances, have had a brilliant career as a teacher. Nightingale's assessment of him as a frustrated would-be factory superintendent does not show much insight into his character, but it may reveal more of her own yearnings and ambitions, projected onto him when she found they were unsuitable for herself. When, at the age of twenty, Nightingale asked if she could study mathematics and began to talk of accomplishing something in the world, her father was uneasy; he seems to have regretted having awakened an appetite for action that could not be fulfilled. There was no useful role for highly educated ladies in Victorian society; Nightingale was already over-qualified for the family duties that awaited her. After much argument, she was allowed to study mathematics under a tutor.

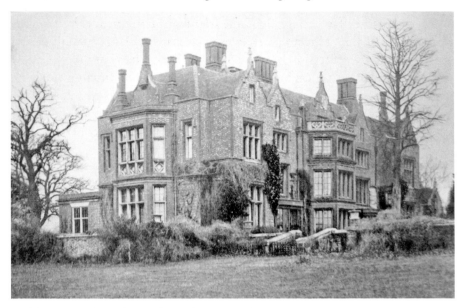

Embley, Hampshire, the Nightingales' winter home.

A certain amount of managerial competence was normal in a lady from the landed class, who was often responsible for managing a large staff of servants and the procurement of supplies. The Nightingale family occupied two large country houses where such skills were needed: Lea Hurst in Derbyshire, and Embley Park, an ornate Elizabethan-style mansion near the New Forest. From July to October each year the family was at Lea Hurst, and from then until March they wintered at Embley. In March the family went to London for the Season, staying usually at the Burlington Hotel in Mayfair. It was an apparently busy life of itinerant socialising, but like many similar Victorian ladies Nightingale recognised the incongruity of such a gilded existence in the midst of poverty, and devoted some of her time to good works in the villages surrounding her father's estates.

The family's energetic socialising brought Nightingale into contact with many of the ruling class, in particular with Lord Palmerston, the future Prime Minister. Palmerston's country house of Broadlands was only a couple of miles from the Nightingales' winter home. Palmerston was a rising young politician in his late thirties when the Nightingales first became his neighbours in 1825. In 1830, when Florence was ten years old, Palmerston became Foreign Secretary. He was later to rise to unheard-of heights of popularity and success as Home Secretary and then Prime Minister during the Crimean War and after. Nightingale's father had seconded the nomination of Lord Palmerston as a successful parliamentary candidate for their local constituency of South Hampshire in the general election that followed passage of the Reform Bill in 1832. Nightingale, barely in her teens, accompanied her father to hear their friend Palmerston speak at public meetings nearby, and pronounced herself satisfied with his foreign policy. William Nightingale unsuccessfully tried to enter parliament himself at the same time, now that reform had made politics compatible with his principles, and his failure was a disappointment to himself and to his daughters. The Palmerstons and the Nightingales often dined together informally. Florence shone in such company, where her erudition made her the conversational equal of the most distinguished men. The notoriously poor quality of the quadrilles that she rendered on the pianoforte may have increased the men's respect for her, as also the fact that she was graceful but fairly plain.

In her twenties, Nightingale formed another close friend in the world of politics. Sidney Herbert, the second son of the Earl of Pembroke, was ten years her senior. As a political contact, Herbert complemented Lord Palmerston to perfection because the two belonged to different parties (Herbert was conservative, Palmerston liberal) and one or the other of them was a Cabinet Minister almost continuously from 1830 to 1865. Each of them, at the time Nightingale first met them, was widely believed to be a future Prime Minister, although Sidney Herbert did not live long enough to achieve it. He and his wife Elizabeth, known as Liz, were a golden couple – he was tall and slim with delicate features, wavy hair, and an irresistibly charming and sincere manner; she was one of the great beauties of the time. They were very wealthy and, like Nightingale, were interested in philanthropy. Sidney did not expect to inherit the family title, so he was able to plan a future in the House of Commons; his older brother, now the Earl, had made an unsuitable marriage to an Italian courtesan and, conveniently for Sidney, had to live abroad, leaving Sidney to occupy the family's stately home at Wilton. Wilton was one of the grandest houses in the country and was not far from the Nightingale mansion at Embley. Sidney had also inherited great wealth independently and was able to live in great style.

Nightingale met the Herberts in Rome through mutual friends in 1847, and she and Sidney had been immediately smitten with each other and talked endlessly together of politics and philanthropy, with Sidney at least pretending to be swayed by Nightingale's extreme left-wing arguments. Gillian Gill, Nightingale's biographer, records that Nightingale dressed up beautifully and had her hair specially done when she dined alone with the Herberts. Sidney and Liz were eventually to be responsible for overcoming the resistance of Nightingale's family to her leaving home.

Nightingale had heard her God call her to his service in 1837, when she was seventeen. In a different society she would no doubt have entered a convent. Seven years later she came to believe that God wanted her to work in hospitals; again, in France or Germany it would have been quite normal for her to become a Sister of Mercy in a religious order dedicated

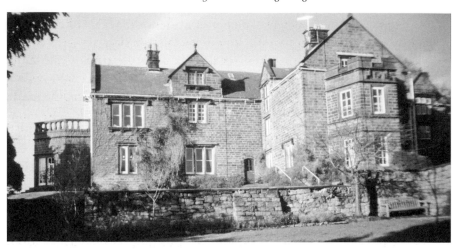

Lea Hurst, Derbyshire. Florence's room is top left, with balcony.

to such work. But in England women were not encouraged to find such outlets for their humanitarian and managerial urges, and Nightingale spent most of her youth dreaming up imaginary scenarios under which she could achieve her goal. In these reveries she escaped from the stifling trivialities of the drawing room to perform heroic humanitarian feats in hospital under the gaze of a beloved masculine leader.

By the time she reached the age of thirty, she was desperate at not having any outlet for her ambitions. In a letter to her parents she claimed that women were driven to madness by the type of imprisonment that she had to suffer: 'I see the numbers of my kind who have gone mad for want of something to do.' The only time she felt satisfied was when she visited the sick poor and taught their children in the village schools near the family home in Derbyshire. 'Oh happy, happy six weeks at Lea Hurst,' she wrote, 'where I had found my business in this world. My heart was filled. My soul was at home. I wanted no other heaven. May God be thanked as He never yet has been thanked for that glimpse of what it is to live.' The attempts of her class to combine social activity with good works repelled her. 'In London there have been the usual amount of Charity Balls, Charity Concerts, Charity Bazaars, whereby people bamboozle their consciences and shut their eyes . . . England is surely the country where luxury has reached its height and poverty its depth.'

There is no question that Nightingale's feelings of social guilt, expressed in the above comments, were genuine. This was not surprising as her family was extremely wealthy, having benefited from the industrial revolution since before even the age of steam. The family woollen mills (still active today) harnessed the water power of the River Derwent, close to the family home at Lea Hurst. From an early age, Nightingale tried to assuage her feelings of guilt by direct action; putting aside the sentimental tales of bandaging dolls and pets there is plenty of evidence that she schemed and plotted to be the one sent to look after any available sick person. Visits to the sick poor by young ladies from wealthy families were not uncommon, along with teaching in village schools, but the difference in Nightingale's case is that these activities were backed by high ambition and an elaborate education. She was probably one of the best educated people in Britain; if women had been allowed into the universities she might still hold the record as the youngest ever graduate, and if women had been allowed into parliament she would have been a very strong candidate for Prime Minister.

Her character would have been more clearly evident in her most personal diaries, which unfortunately disappeared during the Second World War, thirty years after her death. Probably amounting to several hundred thousand words, they made clear the depth of her passionate opposition to the disparity of wealth in Britain and to the prevailing political system. Only a few fragmentary passages survive, printed in O'Malley's 1931 biography. They give glimpses of the young Nightingale's precocity, the agonising guilt that she felt when she became aware of the plight of the poor in Victorian England – amounting almost to a hatred for her own privileged class – and the radical political opinions she developed as she grew to adulthood. Typical of the latter are an argument she had with her new High Tory friend Sidney Herbert in which she claims to have forced Herbert to admit that a republican government would be better for Britain than a monarchy, and her fiery comment when the French were besieging Garibaldi's liberal Roman Republic: 'If I were in Rome, I should be the first to fire the Sistine, turning my head aside, and Michael Angelo would cry 'Well done' as he saw his work destroyed.' The impact of this is all the greater if you read her ecstatic descriptions of the Sistine Chapel from earlier in the same diary. Nightingale is often compared to her admirer Margaret Thatcher, but her politics were more in line with those of the renegade upper-class radical Tony Wedgwood Benn.

Her dearest ambition was to set up and manage hospitals, which at that time were charity institutions for the poor, but whenever the subject was mentioned her mother and sister fainted and had to be revived with smelling salts. She tried to convert to Catholicism and become a nun, proposing to set up a Catholic religious order in England dedicated to training nurses, but the Catholic Church refused her request because Cardinal Manning believed with some reason that she only wanted the support and career path that it gave to its nuns, and not its beliefs. Unlike the Church of Rome, the Church of England had no provision for training women in good works as it did men. There was actually no formal provision in England outside the Roman Catholic Church for training women to do anything at all. Her Unitarian tradition would have made it quite easy for her to convert opportunistically to Catholicism: during the Middle Ages some Unitarians even converted to Judaism to avoid persecution by other Christians.

When, in her twenties, Nightingale first developed an interest in hospitals, her sister Parthenope's anxiety was so intense that her family thought she was unbalanced. Not that they thought Florence's interest in hospitals was normal, either. 'It was as if I had wanted to be a kitchen-maid,' she said in later life. Reluctantly, and carefully hiding the truth from their conventional friends, her parents allowed her to spend some time at an institution where resident 'deaconesses' were trained to care for the poor, at Kaiserswerth in Germany. More respectably, she was encouraged to travel to Egypt and the Continent with family friends. Parthenope was furious at these desertions. According to Nightingale's biographer Ida O'Malley, the tension between the two sisters was partly due to Parthenope's dissatisfaction with her own imprisonment within the family, and her realisation that her more gifted sister's frequent absences increased the workload on Parthenope when it came to caring for the parents and entertaining visitors with intelligent conversation. Florence's description of Parthenope's 'vocation . . . to make holiday for hard working men out of London, who come to enjoy this beautiful place' might have been rather insensitive if one accepts O'Malley's analysis that Parthenope yearned for freedom.

The two sisters could both be expected to have especial difficulties due to their gender, because they had both failed to be the required male heir and their mother could have no more children. The family was a victim of the law of entail, under which their father did not own the family home and the income from its land. He was only the tenant-for-life under the system designed to keep large landed estates intact by preventing their sale and passing them down only through a single male inheritor. Under this system, which survived until the early twentieth century, some estates had not been owned freehold by anybody for hundreds of years. Florence and Parthenope's failure to be male even condemned them and their mother to eviction from the family home when their father died and the male inheritor, possibly not even related, moved in. In addition to thus being punished for being female, any unmarried lady was obliged by social custom to live permanently with her relatives and to care for them and their guests. Hospital work was the kind of thing many upper-class unmarried women yearned for as an alternative to this living death, but they did not have Nightingale's determination or education.

Nightingale railed against the poor quality of a woman's life as compared to a man's in an autobiographical tract she called *Cassandra*, in which she described the middle class unmarried woman as being a slave to her relatives. A woman was always expected to be available to entertain parents or their guests, and could not even retire to her room for study as a man had the right to do. 'Passion, intellect, moral activity,' she wrote, 'these three have never been satisfied in woman'. Nightingale believed that women of her class were trained to suppress their passionate natures, and resorted to fantasy as a result. In her most personal diaries she confessed to being addicted to a what she referred to repeatedly as a loathsome vice, which she called 'dreaming'. This vice, which she describes only in cryptic terms, she called her 'enemy', the 'murderer of her thoughts' and said that it had been with her from a young age. When she was nearly thirty and touring Egypt, she had confessed in her diary to 'dreaming . . . in the very face of God' at one of the temples. The vice made her lethargic and she reports that when young she could temporarily free herself from her addiction by behaving badly. The only actual daydreams that she describes in her autobiographical work *Cassandra* are fantasies which she claims must be common in females of her class, in which the a woman imagines herself working under the command of a dominant male whom she idolises, 'engaged with him in stirring events . . . engaging in romantic dangers with him . . . undergoing unheard-of trials under the observation of some one she has chosen as the companion of her dreams'. This reveals much about Nightingale's early attitude to the opposite sex. Her description of the daydreams, together with her shame at what she calls 'dreaming' but nowhere defines, has led Gillian Gill to propose that her secret 'vice' was masturbation, an activity that adults of the day took enormous pains to eliminate in the young. A medical textbook of 1883 warns doctors that the habit leads to ill-health; 'in the female' it adds, 'the natural feelings are often lost'. The textbook advises medical practitioners to treat the habit with chemotherapy, by thickly bandaging the hands at night or tying them behind the victim's back, and by encouraging early rising, strenuous exercise, and travel. These last three are notable for having been forced on Florence (but not her sister) by her anxious mother. Why adults were so fervently against masturbation when almost all of them must have indulged in it is curious; perhaps they blamed early indulgence in it for all their own shortcomings. If Gill is right, Nightingale was more sexually active than she has been given credit for.

Nightingale admitted in a private note to herself and posterity that one way she could put an end to the 'evil of dreaming' would be to get married. She wrote this when she was twenty-eight and had just rejected a proposal from the opportunistic socialite and fortune-hunter Richard Monckton Milnes. The note was published in 1913 in a heavily censored form and then disappeared. In it, Nightingale said that Milnes might satisfy her 'passional nature', and in the context she must be referring to her sexual needs, but she turned him down because his life of intense socialising did not correspond with her ideal of an idealistic male companion under whose leadership she could accomplish great and dangerous works of philanthropy. She was sensible not to give more weight to the sexual advantages because, as Gill describes in her character sketch, Monckton Milnes was homosexual.

It was the last time she was tempted by marriage. 'I don't agree at all that a woman has no reason for not marrying a good man who asks her,' Nightingale wrote, 'and I don't think Providence does either. I think He has as clearly marked out some to be single women as He has others to be wives.' When she had decided against marriage she knew she had to find her direction: 'Today I am thirty – the age Christ began his Mission. Now no more childish things, no more vain things, no more love, no more marriage. Now, Lord, let me only think of Thy will.'

She realised that her disappointment lay in her failure to make her family understand her ambition to work in a hospital, and this disappointment was caused by her own misguided attempts to enlist their sympathy for her ambitions. 'I must expect no sympathy nor help from them. I have so long craved for their sympathy that I can hardly reconcile myself to this. I have so long struggled to make myself understood . . . I must not even try to be understood. It must be only for fun that I try to make them understand me – because I know that it is impossible.'

The break finally came when she was thirty-two years old. Liz Herbert was on the committee of a charitable institution in Harley Street which looked after sick and impoverished gentlewomen, and she arranged for Nightingale to become the Lady Superintendent. Nightingale was in command at Harley Street from August 1853 to October 1854. Her work consisted largely of organising supplies of goods and services after the recent move from other premises. For example, she terminated the arrangement under which the grocer's boy would call up to three times a day, and instead bought supplies in bulk to be delivered at regular intervals. She brought the dispensary in-house, and reduced the staffing costs. It was similar to the work she was accustomed to at Embley and Lea Hurst, but in a medical context. She attended when surgeons performed operations on the premises, and the only one that she describes ended in failure when the removal of a cataract led to inflammation and blindness. In describing this post-operative complication, at the time Nightingale made no comment about its possible causation by lack of hygiene – a significant omission in the light of her later concerns.

'I am in the heyday of my power,' Nightingale wrote confidently when she was at Harley Street, unaware of the greater things to come. It was not an unrealistic boast: she was at the time probably the most powerful independent woman in Britain if you didn't count the Queen. She chose to rub it in, opposing the committee of her own hospital on the subject of Roman Catholic patients who were rigorously excluded in accordance with the prevailing prejudice. Unless the rules were changed, Nightingale said, she would resign. As a gratuitous slap in the face she demanded that their priests should also be admitted, and for good measure Jews and Muslims together with their rabbis and imams. The horrified committee had no choice but to cave in. Nevertheless, Nightingale was ready to resort to subterfuge to appear orthodox herself; she rented an apartment where she could disappear on Sundays to hide the fact that she was not in church.

When she gave notice after twelve months it was on the grounds that the patients were not interesting enough. They were nearly all either hypochondriacs or incurable cancer sufferers. Nightingale told the committee that she was looking for a position where the medical and surgical treatment offered was more appropriate for instruction of the students in a nursing school. After the first twelve months of her career, therefore, Nightingale had some practical experience of hospital administration, as well as having researched staffing practices in hospitals in Italy, France, Germany, and Egypt. She was looking for a position where she could set up a nursing school in a large London teaching hospital. She and Sidney Herbert (who was by now a Cabinet minister) had already conducted surveys of hospitals, examining the defects in the pay, organisation, and accommodation of nurses. They believed that the obstacle to improving the opportunities for women in nursing was the perception that nurses in hospital were exposed to grave dangers of immorality (sexual harassment, we would call it) and drunkenness. It was these fears, more than the medical horrors, that had made Nightingale's mother oppose her daughter's initial attempts to attach herself a hospital. Overcoming them would enable other women with less powerful friends to escape from the trap that Nightingale had been born in.

Her experience with supplies and her knowledge of best practice in managing female staff in hospital made Nightingale an obvious choice to lead a party of nurses to the Crimean War. So did her mental outlook. She had a sort of towering optimism and confidence, based not just on self-esteem but on a deep spiritual belief that the universe is fundamentally on the side of mankind. She was even able to look back on her long imprisonment in the family, immediately after she had made the break, and see that it had served its purpose. It had been a gestation period, while she learned how to create herself individually as mankind must create itself collectively. She wrote to her father on her thirty-second birthday, thanking him for his support in breaking free: 'I am glad to think that my youth is past, and rejoice that it never, never can return – that time of follies and bondage, of unfulfilled hopes and disappointed inexperience, when a man possesses nothing, not even himself. When I speak of disappointed inexperience I accept it, not only as inevitable, but as the beautiful arrangement of Infinite Wisdom, which cannot create us gods, but which will not create us animals, and therefore wills mankind to create mankind by their own experience.' This philosophy of 'mankind creating mankind' was a Unitarian position. At this time, Nightingale tried to explain the philosophy in a monograph addressed *To the Artizans of England*. She had entered into religious discussions with some of the working men in the villages surrounding Lea Hurst, and found that they had no respect for traditional religion, so she wrote this monograph hoping to convert them to a rational religious philosophy devised for the manufacturing age. The artisans of Derbyshire must have had a rather pessimistic view of human nature, because her 1852 tract is a justification of the belief that human nature is innately good, despite the historical evidence to the contrary. Although the history of human nature appears to be a history of evil, Nightingale finds the solution to this problem in the explanation that our awareness that the past is evil is precisely what makes our nature good: we recognise improvement.

Her tract shows that in 1852 she had already studied the work of the Belgian statistician and social scientist Adolphe Quetelet, although she does not mention him by name. She says that the number of murders in a particular social group can now be foretold, and the variations between groups can be used to find out and alter the circumstances that cause a high murder rate. This was a reference to Quetelet's approach of using statistics to explore social trends. The comprehensive registration of births, marriages, and deaths which started in England in 1837 allowed socio-economic statistics to be collected for the first time. The proportion of people able to sign their name on a marriage certificate, for example, gave a crude index of the education level in a particular area, and it soon became apparent that crime was lower in counties with higher education, even when the level of income was the same. Such evidence was eagerly seized upon by social improvers.

There is no evidence that Nightingale at that time considered statistics useful for day-to-day hospital management or for public health. Her 1852 tract also shows that her interest in disease was rather superficial. She writes in the *Artizans* that, contrary to popular belief encouraged by the clergy, cholera is not God's way of punishing sin, rather it is 'incident on certain states of body under certain circumstances'. By the time she went to the war two years later, she had begun to associate cholera with lack of cleanliness.

After the war, Nightingale revised *To the Artizans of England* and incorporated it into a much longer book entitled *Suggestions for Thought*. We shall see in due course that a comparison of the two texts shows how the war and its aftermath changed her ideas. Meanwhile, it is remarkable that in 1852 Nightingale already counsels her artisans that, just as mankind must do badly in order to do better, so must individuals inevitably make serious mistakes. 'A healthy moral nature, having on an occasion erred,' according to Nightingale, 'should regret the error, even though it was inevitable in God's scheme of things, but should not feel remorse.' Two years later, a few weeks before leading a party of nurses to the Crimean War, Nightingale commented in a letter to her sister on the unfortunate case of a Mother Superior who accidentally poisoned one of her nuns: 'your mistakes are a part of God's plan.' It seems that she believed that God needed people with good intentions who were prepared to take risks. This may have been a more common belief in those days of personal philanthropy than it is today. It was to stand her in good stead.

In October 1854, one month after Nightingale gave her notice at Harley Street, a crisis erupted in the new general hospitals that the British Army had established in Scutari, at a safe distance from the war zone in the Crimea. The first important battle was in September 1854, and when the wounded arrived at the hospital they found it bare of supplies. *The Times* began criticising the lack of equipment, even of bandages, at Scutari: 'When the wounded are placed in the spacious building where we were led to believe that everything was ready which would ease their pain or facilitate their recovery, it is found that the commonest appliances of a work-house sick ward are wanting.'

The world's most powerful industrial nation was filling its steamships with unheard-of quantities of supplies for despatch to the hospitals – bandages by the ton, and 15,000 pairs of sheets according to Herbert – but for some reason none of it was arriving at the right place. It was ending up in Bulgaria, which the army had left months previously, or supplies destined for Constantinople were going to the Crimea instead. Some supplies were even being brought back to England because nobody would take responsibility for them at the destination. Meanwhile the officials in charge at Scutari were telling the Cabinet that nothing was wrong – according to them there were no shortages.

At the same time the male orderlies who were supposed to look after the patients had been badly recruited and proved incapable. Comparisons were drawn with the superior female nursing provided by nuns in the French hospitals. 'Why have we no Sisters of Charity?' cried *The Times* plaintively. It seemed an ideal opportunity to try out the new kind of highly disciplined and organised nursing proposed by Nightingale. At the time, Sidney Herbert was trying to find a way to use his position in the Cabinet to solve the problems of female nursing in English teaching hospitals and create career opportunities for people like his friend Florence Nightingale. If it could be shown that a party of English nurses could survive contact with a horde of soldiers in the field, then the horrors of a London teaching hospital and its dissolute medical students would no longer prevent the introduction of respectable women into an environment where they could be taught to be of real use. It was inevitable that Sidney Herbert and his wife should conceive the idea of sending Florence Nightingale to the East.

Sidney Herbert's job in the Cabinet was a junior one. It created so much confusion in managing the war that it was abolished four months later when the government was overthrown largely because of this confusion. His title was Secretary at War; the job was so unimportant that it had not always carried a seat in the Cabinet. A different Cabinet minister, the Duke of Newcastle, was responsible for operational conduct of the war, and Sidney Herbert's job was to oversee only the finances of the army. He used his position to persuade the Duke of Newcastle that his friend Florence Nightingale was the only independent advisor who understood hospital management. The Duke of Newcastle therefore delegated the management of the hospital to Herbert, and allowed him to invite Nightingale to lead a party of nurses to Scutari. Herbert's published instructions reveal that he was sending Nightingale to the war to promote the idea of female hospital nursing as well as to serve the sick. 'If this succeeds, an enormous amount of good will be done, now, and to persons deserving everything at our hands, and a prejudice will have been broken through, and precedent established, which will multiply the good to all time.' Nightingale and Herbert believed that draconian discipline could solve the problems of sexual harassment and could also stop the nurses incapacitating themselves with alcohol.

Nightingale's local rank was to be Superintendent of Female Nursing, but the skill at hospital management which she had demonstrated at Harley Street allowed Herbert to give her secret instructions, not announced to the newspapers, to inform the Cabinet of any non-nursing problems she encountered, and even to take direct action to resolve them. The government was prepared to give Nightingale unlimited authority to spend money on its behalf, and Herbert appeared to have solved the problems of Scutari at a stroke. And so, on 21 October 1854, aged only thirty-four and at the head of a band of thirty-eight nurses, Florence Nightingale set off for Constantinople on a P&O steamer under the instruction and observation of her handsome hero Sidney Herbert. It was as if one of the heroic daydreams of her youth had come true.

CHAPTER TWO

At War

Turkey had declared war on Russia in 1853, after Russia invaded some of the European provinces of Turkey's Ottoman Empire. The war divided opinion along party political lines in Britain. Reactionary conservatives (including Prince Albert, Queen Victoria's husband) believed in autocratic government and in the divine right of Christian kings like Tsar Nicholas and so supported the Tsar in his crusade against Turkey. They believed that Turkey had no business occupying provinces in Europe and looked forward to Russia's reconquest of Constantinople, the ancient seat of the Christian church. The Tsar, relying on some earlier conversations with a more conservative British government, believed that Britain would not oppose his dismemberment of the Ottoman Empire. But by 1853, Britain was governed by a conservative/liberal coalition, and the liberal popular mood was very anti-Russian because of the Tsar's repressive and expansionist policies. Under successive Russian Tsars, the Empire had expanded dramatically into Europe by conquering Poland, the Ukraine, Byelorussia, the Baltic States, and parts of Sweden, the Caucasus, and European Turkey. Karl Marx, exiled in London, was already calling Russia 'the prison of nations', and liberals throughout Europe were concerned that Russia might conquer the continent's few remaining independent countries and add them to its totalitarian Empire. Conservatives, on the other hand, thought that a totalitarian and theocratic Russia was just what was needed for Europe: a force for stability.

Eventually the conservative element in Britain's coalition grudgingly agreed to a declaration of war on Russia in March 1854, six months after the Turks had done so, because they were persuaded that Russia's growing sea power threatened the dominance of the Royal Navy. France joined in on Britain' side and the only two industrialised and well-armed countries in Europe sent a large expeditionary force to eject Russia from the Turkish provinces. The Turks pushed out the Russians without foreign help, however, and the question then arose whether the war was over. France and Britain, with the approval of the majority of European states including

Sweden, Spain, Italy, and the Austrian Empire, decided to continue the war by invading a suitable territory on the periphery of the Russian Empire and thus beginning the liberation of the captive states. The Crimea, which Russia had conquered from Turkey within living memory, was the obvious choice; the region appealed to British conservatives because it contained the huge naval base of Sebastopol, which was the source of their only real anxiety about Russia.

Britain, France, and Turkey invaded the Crimea in September 1854 and soon met and defeated an army that had occupied what the Russians had believed was an impregnable position on high ground at the River Alma outside Sebastopol. The British and French common soldiers displayed great initiative at this first battle although (or perhaps because) their senior officers had made no tactical plan. Neither was there any real plan for treating the wounded; the outcry in the British press over the shabby treatment of the wounded after the Alma was the start of the process that led to Florence Nightingale being sent to war.

The Crimea is a lozenge-shaped peninsula that hangs down from the top of the Black Sea. The entrance to the Black Sea from the Mediterranean is near Constantinople (now Istanbul) through the narrow strait of the Bosphorus about 300 miles south of the Crimea. The Bosphorus is about 20 miles long, from 1 to 3 miles wide, and flows between wooded cliffs backed by distant mountains. This unusual geographic feature divides Europe from Asia, European Turkey from Anatolian Turkey, and the old part of Constantinople known as Stamboul from the suburb of Uskudar on the Anatolian shore. The British name for Uskudar was Scutari, and in Scutari, standing on a clifftop, is the vast Turkish barracks which the British in 1854 decided to borrow for use as a military hospital.

From the windows of the Scutari Barrack Hospital, the view down over the Bosphorus to the old city of Stamboul was superb. According to Florence Nightingale, who had travelled to some exotic spots in the Mediterranean, it was the best view in the world. She liked to watch the sun set directly behind the domes and minarets of Stamboul. Scutari itself was a quiet backwater whose empty spaces, formerly an assembly point for the caravans that set off on the pilgrimage to Mecca, had been deserted by the camels and not yet invaded by the motor-car.

The British occupied the Scutari barracks early in 1854, using it at first as a depot on the way to Bulgaria and later as a hospital. It was only after the invasion of the Crimea and the battle of the Alma in September that large numbers of patients began to arrive there by ship from the Crimea. When Florence Nightingale arrived at the beginning of November 1854, Scutari was already full and more patients were arriving daily.

The Army Medical Department staff were not pleased to see her. Communication with London took two weeks in each direction, and

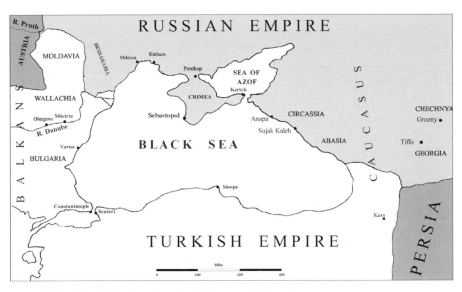

Map of the Black Sea showing the Crimea and Scutari.

although they could see that she and her nurses had authorisation to work there, the doctors themselves had no instructions on how to employ them and considered their intrusion to be a sign of lack of confidence in their own abilities. They therefore refused to give her or her nurses any instructions. Nightingale could have gone to work immediately, if only feeding the patients – many of her nurses were nuns who had experience of nursing without medical supervision. But she refused to work or to allow her nurses to work on this basis. Sidney Herbert had said she would act 'in the strictest subordination to the Chief Medical Officer', and that was what she insisted on doing. She wanted to underline the fact that she was a functionary of the state – a revolutionary status for a woman – not a charity worker. Dr Menzies, the Chief Medical Officer at Scutari, had the Army Medical Department rank of Deputy Inspector General, which was officially equivalent to the combatant rank of lieutenant-colonel. Superintendent Nightingale, therefore, occupied a position in the military hierarchy equivalent to a major. Towards the end of the war, Nightingale was promoted to General Superintendent of the Female Nursing Establishment of the Military Hospitals of the Army, reporting to Sir John Hall. He held the rank of Inspector General of Hospitals, which was equivalent to brigadier-general, so his subordinate, General Superintendent Nightingale, was entitled to think herself as being on the level of a full colonel. Unlike male officers, she did not have a written commission and is not in the Army List, but it is important to realise that she was not just an up-market camp-follower. She was a part of the military hierarchy, and the fact was not welcome to those above her.

She therefore threatened her nurses with dismissal if they attended a patient without instructions from a doctor. The instructions not being forthcoming, Florence Nightingale and her unhappy band sat for three days and four nights in their quarters making bandages and occasionally treating a sick civilian. On the fourth day there was a surge of arrivals from the Crimea: wounded from Inkerman and sick men suffering from the onset of winter, evacuated because of the continued Russian threat to the British beachhead at Balaclava. The doctors, overwhelmed, asked the nurses to help in the wards and Nightingale told the women to get busy. This incident has given Nightingale a reputation for 'subservience' to the medical profession. If insisting on receiving orders from doctors who refuse to give them – and winning the contest – is subservience then her reputation is deserved. It was evidently the kind of subservience that the Army Medical Department did not relish. One can understand why, because taking orders gave her and her nurses the right enjoyed by every British subordinate to officially question those orders. For example, Nightingale asked a male orderly to give a patient a hot water bottle because his feet were cold; the orderly, a corporal, said that he could not do so without a doctor's approval. She insisted on sending for the overworked Duty Medical Officer who made it obvious that he should not have been troubled for such a trivial matter. Most nurses would have been overawed and would have avoided causing such trouble in future, but Nightingale wrote a politely sarcastic letter to the senior surgeon in charge of the ward, ridiculing the regulations. If this was subservience, it had a sting in the tail.

Within three weeks of her arrival there were 2,300 patients in the Barrack Hospital. The hospital supplies still had not materialised. Shiploads of chamber pots had disappeared into thin air; dysentery was rife among the prostrate casualties. There were no basins, no towels, and no soap. Only thirty patients a day could be cleaned in the few hip baths available. The officials in charge of the stores were hoarding the supplies they had, and the medical officers were so frightened of making trouble that they refused to write requisitions and claimed that they had everything they needed. Nightingale and a Mr MacDonald from *The Times* scoured the bazaars of Constantinople for basic necessities, often using money given by the readers of that newspaper instead of government funds.

Ten days after Nightingale arrived in Constantinople, there was a hurricane in the Black Sea. Dozens of British supply ships sank, including a modern steamship that contained most of the army's winter clothing and tons of supplies for Scutari that had not been unloaded when the ship called there because they lay underneath the ammunition destined for the Crimea further on. The army camped outside Sebastopol crouched helpless as the wind tore away the tents from around them in the night. When dawn broke, the men found themselves marooned on a bleak plateau 6 miles from the only harbour through which supplies could be landed. The Russians had captured the road from the harbour to the camp during the battle of Balaclava in October, and the only way to bring in supplies was now over a muddy track up the mountainside. It seemed as if even Brunel's marvellous modern steamship the *Great Britain*, one of the wonders of the world, could not help the British Army now. The world's most advanced industrial state could not protect its troops from the onslaught of winter. A fortune in supplies piled up in the tiny port of Balaclava. An opposition MP pointed out in the House that the Minister of War had transported a full complement of supplies a distance of 3,000 miles, but unfortunately the distance to the camp was 3,006.

There were no more battles until the spring, but the men kept coming into Nightingale's hospital. Scurvy, dysentery, and frostbite were spreading through the camp on the plateau above Sebastopol. Throughout the winter, a steady stream of sick men trickled down the hillside to Balaclava harbour, mostly on mules provided and driven by the efficient French ambulance corps. In the harbour they were loaded slowly onto ships for a

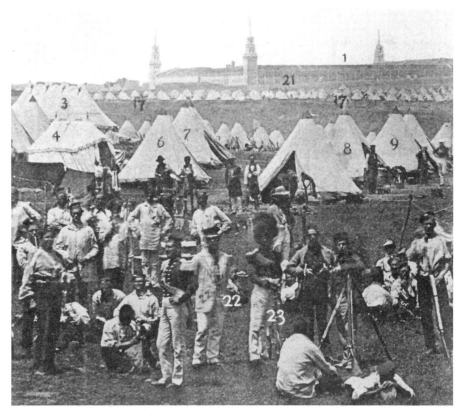

The camp of the Grenadier Guards at Scutari, in front of the Barrack Hospital where some of them were later to die.

voyage of several days across the Black Sea to Scutari. Many died on the track, in the harbour, or on the transports, and others died while waiting to be brought ashore in small boats at Scutari, where the ruined landing pier was unusable. The survivors staggered or were carried up to Florence Nightingale's Barrack Hospital.

The hospital was an enormous rectangular building of three floors with a tower at each corner, built around an enclosed quadrangle or parade ground. On each floor, a single corridor ran around all four sides of the building. The corridor was on the inside, next to the enclosed quadrangle, which was between 4 and 5 metres wide with a high ceiling. Leading off the corridor on the outside of the building were barrack rooms used as wards, more than a hundred of them on each floor and each about 7 metres square. In these wards a low wooden bench barely ankle high ran around the room, upholstered and stuffed with uncomfortably hard material. On the side of the room next to the corridor there was a wooden gallery below the ceiling. The floors of the rooms were of wood, often rotten; the corridors were paved with broken unglazed tiles.

At first, Nightingale was the only female allowed inside the hospital at night. She used to walk the length of the corridors before going to bed, a distance of more than 800 yards around the four sides of the rectangular building. Then she would go to the other floors and walk a similar distance again, in the dim half light of crude oil-dip lamps. The corridor was lined with beds – most of them simple straw-filled mattresses on the tile floor. The men lay with their heads towards the wall, with only a metre or so separating their feet from the opposite mattress and barely half that separating each mattress from the one next to it. In the barrack rooms the separation was similar, and if every available space was taken the whole building could theoretically have held around 3,000 patients. At its peak there was a patient population of 2,500. The death rate was then at its peak, too – up to seventy in a single day. Few soldiers could be found strong enough to carry a load, and Turkish labourers carried away the corpses as well as bringing the new arrivals up from the landing pier. At night the patients hardly ever spoke; they lay in deathlike silence as Nightingale passed alone between the endless lines of beds in the corridor. Most of them had been admitted suffering from sickness; those wounded in battle were more often sent to another hospital nearby.

During the first four months after Nightingale arrived, there was hardly any ventilation in the hospital. The windows were small and were shut tight against the cold, with broken panes stuffed with rags. Heating was by iron stoves whose chimneys led out through holes in the windows. The wall separating the corridor from the rooms prevented any possibility of a through draught. The filth and infestation in the wards and corridors cannot be adequately described.

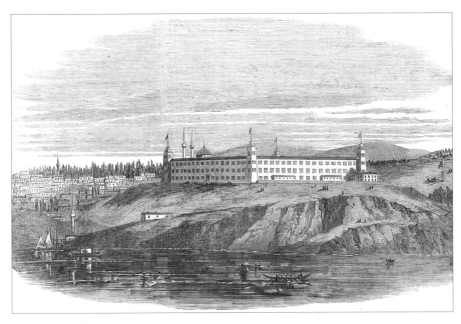

The Barrack Hospital, Scutari.

Either the medical staff or Nightingale herself initially barred nurses from the hospital at night. Some doctors refused to have nurses on their corridors or rooms even during the day, but after a while, some of the medical officers wanted nurses to help them visit patients during the night and the prohibition was relaxed. Those medical officers who preferred a callous approach had ways to justify it. One was the fact that the soldiers were there by individual choice. Unlike those of Continental Europe where conscription was almost universal, the British Army was a volunteer one.

Nightingale's letters home show that she believed that the common soldier was being deprived of the basic necessities of life in hospital by lazy or incompetent officials. According to her, artificial shortages went unreported by frightened medical officers whose career could be ruined by writing requisitions that they knew would not be filled. Patients were left in the care of drunken orderlies who were often malingering soldiers, thieves avid for the savings of the dying, or pensioners who had foolishly volunteered to come out of retirement to accompany the army and were rapidly succumbing to disease and delirium tremens. Nightingale and her nurses quickly identified the doctors who were susceptible to moral pressure and enrolled them in a conspiracy to cheat the lazy officials and get more food for their patients. Nightingale did the same thing on a broader and more organised scale. She was impressed by the meekness and simplicity of the common soldier in the hour of his trial. 'I have never been able to join in the popular cry about the recklessness, sensuality, and

helplessness of the soldiers. Give them suffering and they will bear it . . .
Give them work and they will do it. I would rather have to do with the
army than with any other class I have ever attempted to serve.'

Her innovations were at first of a very basic nature. Ten days after
arriving, she wrote to a surgeon she admired in England telling him: 'I am
getting a screen now for the amputations, for when one poor fellow, who
is to be amputated tomorrow, sees his comrade today die under the knife it
makes an impression – and diminishes his chance.' Before that, the surgeons
operated in full view of the other patients in the ward, because there was
no operating room. Nightingale's screen, despite her optimism, made no
difference to the mortality from amputations which she later estimated at
82 per cent. But it may have done something for human dignity.

The army doctors, most of them young and very inexperienced, reacted
to the horrors that surrounded them in different ways. The nurses found
that even the kindly doctors became exasperated and unreasonable when
the newly arrived patients died in such large numbers. A nurse reported
that one of the doctors seldom appeared in the wards at all but remained
in his own quarters, smoking. Another junior surgeon wrote furious letters
home criticising the nurses, including Nightingale. He claimed that she
had made a patient wait for fifteen minutes because she insisted on being
present at all operations. Worse, he claimed that Nightingale dressed
the wounds of a soldier while his genitals were exposed in a way that
'must have been hurtful to his feelings'. This young surgeon wrote of
Nightingale: 'She may be a lady, but I don't think she has the modesty

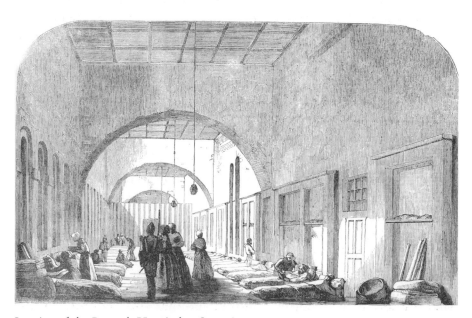

Interior of the Barrack Hospital at Scutari.

of anyone deserving to be a woman.' His letter caused consternation at home, and was suppressed by his superiors; later he died at Scutari, and was nursed by Nightingale personally.

Body lice swarmed on the emaciated patients, 'as thick as the letters on a page of print', and the genitals of a wounded soldier who had been months in the trenches without washing would not have been a pretty sight. Nor would the wounds themselves, but Nightingale sometimes described them with something like admiration in her letters home: 'The Surgeons pass on to the next, an excision of the shoulder-joint – beautifully performed and going on well – bullet lodged just in the head of the joint, and fracture starred all round.'

Her sister Parthenope became Florence's enthusiastic public relations officer in England during the war. She lobbied home officials on Florence's side in her disputes with other officials in the East. She also copied out Florence's letters home for wide circulation, but she was careful to suppress the descriptions of wounds and other aspects of Florence's perverse habit of dwelling on things that ordinary people did not find interesting. A senior army officer who visited Scutari was appalled that Nightingale 'seems to delight in witnessing surgical operations, with arms folded.'

Some nurses who had thought that they would contribute to the men's recovery wanted to go home when they found it was not to be. Most of them, though, were satisfied to make the men's last hours more pleasant, to give them a little dream of home before the end. They schemed to extract more food from the officials, convinced that at least this prolonged life. When these schemes failed, the nurses were sometimes so distressed that the dying patients had to comfort them. The nurses scared the visiting wife of the British Ambassador by telling her that the doctors were deliberately starving the patients and the gullible Lady Stratford began to send up delicacies. One nurse was carrying Lady Stratford's latest delivery when a callous doctor asked her contemptuously: 'Are you giving calves' foot jelly to *soldiers*?' The nurse defiantly replied: 'To dying men.'

The nurses were traumatised by the high death rate. 'It seems strange that we could witness such scenes and sufferings calmly, but to us and to the poor sufferers there seemed granted a calm and quiet temper and a sort of stunned feeling, because had we realised all their sad sufferings we could not have borne it. Daily we missed some pale face we had just learned to know and love, and who loved us, and daily we watched some solitary pilgrim pass peacefully through the dark waters of death. In the course of a few days all who had been entrusted to us had gone, and were succeeded by others who equally seemed doomed to die.'

Nightingale wrote dozens of letters to bereaved families: 'Dear Mrs. Hunt, I grieve to be obliged to inform you that your son died in this hospital on Sunday last. His complaint was chronic dysentery – he sank

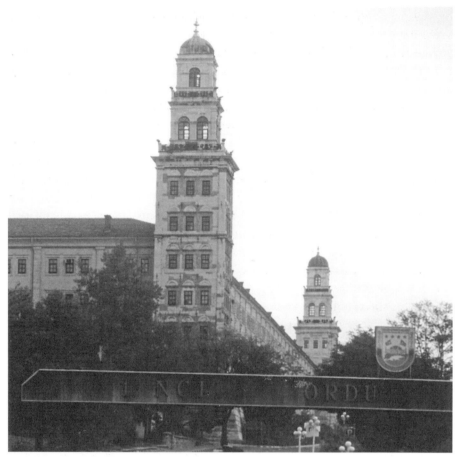

The tower at the Barrack Hospital where Nightingale had her quarters. The other tower in the background houses the museum.

gradually from weakness, without much suffering. Everything was done that was possible to keep up his strength. He was fed every half hour with the most nourishing things he could take, and when there was anything he had a fancy for, it was taken to him immediately. He sometimes asked for oranges and grapes, which quenched his thirst, and which he had, whenever he wished for them. He was very grateful for whatever was done for him, and very patient.'

The nurses could not understand *why* the men were dying; they suspected that the death rate at Scutari was worse than elsewhere, and sought explanations. A nurse wrote: 'The amputations which took place in the hospital were, as far as I knew, mostly unsuccessful. The patient sunk and died under the operation, or soon after it, while those amputated on the field mostly recovered. The reason of this was, I think, that on the field the men were in the full vigour of life, and able to bear the pain and exhaustion, while those operated on in the hospital were worn out by suffering.'

The Angel of Death was always efficient. One night two nurses were told to stay up to look after eight patients whose lives were in danger, with instructions to call two more nurses to replace them at midnight. But the second shift was never needed; all eight patients died well ahead of schedule, 'and when all were at rest we returned to our quarters and went to bed'. The nurses were haunted by the experience for the rest of their lives. 'One lad asked me for a drink, and then to read to him,' remembered one, 'and then at his request I wrote for him to his friends in Oxford. He said "It has pleased the Lord to take my comrade in the night, but I am spared a little longer," but in passing in the evening I spoke to him and, getting no answer, I found he was gone. He asked me to kiss him before he died, and I am sorry I did not.' These must have been very difficult words for this woman to write many years later.

One night the same young nurse followed Nightingale to the dead-house, where the day's corpses from her hospital lay. 'It was an awful place to visit at any time, and as I waited at the door and saw Miss Nightingale calmly uncover the faces of the dead, and look on them as they lay far from wife or mother in that dreary place, it seemed strange to see one so frail, graceful, and refined standing at the dead of night alone amid such sad scenes of mortality.' Nightingale was going to have reason to remember those faces of the dead.

Six weeks after her arrival at Scutari at the head of her party of thirty-eight nurses, another party arrived containing 'ladies' as well as working-class nurses whom Nightingale had not agreed to receive. She was furious with Sidney Herbert for sending them and threatened to resign. She did not think she could impose discipline by herself on such a large number of women, especially because there was not enough room in the hospital to lodge them all. Putting women in lodgings outside the hospital would make it even more difficult to stop them fraternising with the soldiers or getting intoxicated. 'The ladies come out to get married, and the nurses come out to get drunk' she wrote. She slept with the key to the nurses' quarters under her pillow.

Lord Raglan wanted to bring the extra nurses to the Crimea to staff new hospitals closer to the front. The risk that the Russians would overrun the port at Balaclava now seemed more remote, and it would therefore be safe to open hospitals there. But Nightingale opposed Raglan's wishes. One of the newly arrived nurses, Elizabeth Davis, went to see Nightingale and told her she wanted to go to the Crimea because she would be more useful there. Her description of Nightingale's hostile response is remarkably vivid: '"Before I go any further," said Miss Nightingale, "I want to impress one thing particularly on your mind. If you do go to the Crimea, you go against my will". This she repeated over and over again. I persevered in my intention of going to Balaclava, and she observed, "Well, Mrs Davis, I can't let you go without someone to over-look you. If you do go," she added, joining her open hands sideways together, and then forcibly dividing them and spreading out her arms by her sides, "I have done with you and your new superintendent *entirely*".'

This shows that it was not for lack of a superintendent that Nightingale did not want the nurses to go to the Crimea. She obviously did not want to delegate that role for one reason or another. Even her supporters said that she found it difficult to delegate responsibility during the early months of the war. There was also the fact that her authority in the hospitals in the Crimea was not clearly defined. Her original letter of instructions said that she was in charge of nursing at hospitals in Turkey – and at that time there were no others. Eventually the War Office sent an order clarifying her status as General Superintendent of the hospitals outside Turkey as well, but before then she was naturally concerned that trying to supervise nurses in the Crimea would lead to arguments with the medical authorities there.

In the first winter of the war, the only way Nightingale could see of controlling nurses was by centralising both nurses and patients physically under her gaze. Other nurses 'deserted to the front' like Elizabeth Davis; unsupervised and disowned by Nightingale, they showed extraordinary heroism and devotion. They included Jane Shaw Stewart, Mary Seacole, and the unruly Martha Clough who disobeyed all the Nightingale rules and installed herself in a primitive regimental field hospital where she could indulge her weakness for claret to the full.

Rather than encourage new hospitals nearer the front, Nightingale acted to increase the size of her own hospital by restoring some dilapidated parts of the building. When the construction work ran into difficulties because the British Ambassador declined to fund it, she paid for it herself. She increased the approved capacity from 1,220 to 1,600 beds, though the actual number of patients was higher and the hospital was permanently overcrowded. Nightingale knew that she could act on her own initiative like this because of the secret instructions she had received from Sidney Herbert, which required her to act when necessary beyond her public job description as Superintendent of Female Nurses. To rehabilitate and furnish additional wards in the hospital, however, she needed some cooperation from the medical authorities. They were still resentful of her power and unwilling to authorise any decisive action because departmental responsibilities were so confused. The only person to go along with her plans did so because he was in love with her.

CHAPTER THREE

Stirring Events, Romantic Dangers

The Superintendent was First Class Staff Surgeon Alexander MacGrigor, a bachelor in his mid-forties who had been an army surgeon for twenty years. His letters from Scutari to his brother-in-law in Scotland are preserved in the British Library, and include two notes written to him by Florence Nightingale. They have not been published before and show that Nightingale could be a more friendly, warm, cooperative, and confiding colleague than appears from the bulk of her correspondence. They also show how free she was from what we imagine to be conventional Victorian constraints on women. One might be excused for thinking that she would have been constantly chaperoned at Scutari as she was at home, which would make it hard for her to conduct confidential business with her male colleagues, but this was not the case.

Within two weeks of her arrival, Nightingale and MacGrigor had become close sympathisers in the struggle to alleviate the plight of their patients. The newly arrived nurses, he wrote to his brother-in-law, 'are under the charge of a Miss Nightingale, a lady of very large fortune and one of the most amiable creatures on earth. Her sole object to me appears to [be to] relieve the sufferings of her fellow-beings and she certainly spares neither trouble nor expense. She is in my quarters almost any hour of the day'. And after they had together rebuilt the dilapidated wards: 'Miss Nightingale is one of the kindest and most delightful of women. She and I are very great friends. I speak to her as if I had known her all my life.'

MacGrigor might have been exaggerating a little, but not much. Two months after her arrival, she invited herself to his quarters: 'I would like to see you for half an hour before the post goes out tomorrow, but not while Mr Macdonald is there. If you are not well enough, will you tell me and I will come to you either this evening or tomorrow morning? Florence Nightingale.'

Despite their efforts, at this time the situation in the hospital had become desperate. The terrible weather at the battlefront was taking its toll and sick soldiers poured into Scutari. In the single month of January

1855, 10 per cent of the entire British Army in the East died of sickness in the hospitals, many of them in Nightingale's arms. In her efforts to provide for the patients, Nightingale became so dependant on MacGrigor that she feared what would happen if someone were appointed over his head; as a Staff Surgeon he was very junior to be managing such a large establishment. She wrote to Herbert asking that he be promoted to Deputy Inspector General of Hospitals two years earlier than his seniority indicated. Given the hostility and jealousy of some of the other medical staff, this was bound to lead to ill-feeling. But Herbert complied, and let Nightingale break the news:

> I have the very great honour to congratulate you on your promotion. Mr. Herbert says 'Dr. MacGrigor's promotion will go out to him next week'. You had better, however, not know it, as it will be attributed to you [?me] and there will be jealousy and dissatisfaction. Pray therefore do not mention this even to Mrs. Bracebridge [her closest confidant]. It is the only pleasant news I had yesterday. Florence Nightingale.

Single British men in foreign lands are renowned for falling in love with any woman from home who crosses their path, particularly nurses. It is hardly surprising that MacGrigor by this time had fallen for the woman whose warmth, humanity, fortune, and ability to secure promotion were a dream come true. He proudly sent Nightingale's congratulatory note to his brother-in-law and sister and became ever more hopeful:

> There was one (whose note I enclose) stuck closer to me than a brother and on her excellent and well regulated mind and judgment I perseveringly and undauntingly exerted and brought into operation ways and means for the relief of our poor sick and wounded soldiers . . . How I should like to <u>marry</u> that dear woman. £30,000 with estates in Hampshire and Derbyshire but pray do not breathe this to anyone . . . I love her for the deeds she has done, and I really believe she loves me. She will do anything for me I ask. I must bide my time. I may some day on my return to England ask a more delicate and important question than can be propounded here – and volumes might be written on what has already transpired. She is pretty! Ladylike, amiable, and possessing a very large fortune.

Did Nightingale see MacGrigor as the future 'companion of her dreams', the philanthropist with whom she could 'engage in stirring events and romantic dangers, undergoing unheard-of trials under his observation'? Probably not, and in MacGrigor's letters he makes no indication that any sweet nothings had actually passed between them, although he was

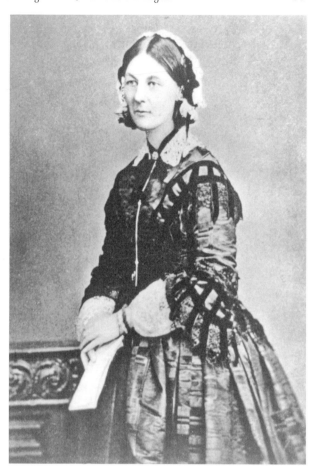

Florence Nightingale
in 1856.

undoubtedly boastful and indiscreet enough to say if they had. The warm
note of congratulation from Nightingale does not show any sentimental
attachment on her part, and yet . . . it *is* rather indiscreet. It would have
been more appropriate for Nightingale to have revealed such sensitive
news verbally. By this time she knew that she was famous, and that if
the note became public it would be embarrassing. So at the very least the
written note appears to be a memento for him and a token of absolute
trust as well as a communication.

   Her earlier fantasies of a philanthropic male companion must have
fuelled her close relationship with MacGrigor even if she did not see him
as the prospective partner. Did he tell Nightingale that he had fathered a
daughter, Isabella, by a young woman shortly before he was posted to the
Scutari? There was no question of his marrying the woman, who seems to
have been a classic 'victim of a rich man's whim' as the song has it, though
he did instruct his brother-in-law to contribute to her support: 'I hope
you are not forgetting my little article at York. She tells me that the little

thing grows apace and a pretty child – I must not act ill towards it.' Such was the patronising male attitude of the times, but at least it shows that MacGrigor would have been more likely to satisfy Nightingale's 'passional nature' than Monckton Milnes, even if his financial motives were no better.

MacGrigor intended to take ship for the journey of several days across the Black Sea to visit the battlefront in the Crimea, though he had less creditable reasons than Nightingale: 'I am thinking of going to the Crimea for a short time with Miss Nightingale if it is only to see the state of things and get the Crimea medal. She is anxious that I accompany her.'

She may have been too quick to trust MacGrigor, because an article appeared in a British newspaper in the spring of 1855 suggesting that the two of them were going to marry. Possibly something had leaked out as a result of his indiscreet letters to his family. Mrs Bracebridge, the close family friend who had come out to Scutari with her husband to help Nightingale, referred to the potential inconvenience caused by this newspaper article when giving the clearest possible indication that Nightingale was accustomed to being alone with MacGrigor and presumably with other male officials: 'She must see a great deal of him and . . . it will be so awkward to receive him alone.'

He did not go to the Crimea with Nightingale, and their trusting relationship cooled. The newspaper article presumably did not help, and his notoriety for having been promoted through favouritism irked him and made him less willing to go out on a limb for her. After a few months she described him as incompetent. MacGrigor died, with three other doctors, in a cholera outbreak at Scutari in November 1855. It is pleasing to relate that his sister and brother-in-law invited Isabella MacGrigor Moyser, his daughter by Mary Moyser of York, into their home near Aberdeen and continued to supplement the mother's income from working in an asylum. The file ends with Mary's polite and confident letters to them, in which she made excellent use of her basic literacy. 'Sorry to give you the trouble so often but if you could let me have the money 2 a year I should be very much a blidge to you. I am now living as a atendant on the in-Sain.'

In late January of 1855, when Nightingale had been in the East for nearly three months, the government in which her old friend Sidney Herbert was a Cabinet Minister fell from power when the House of Commons voted to conduct a public enquiry into its mismanagement of the war. Lord Palmerston, who had been Home Secretary in the disgraced government, formed a new government with himself as Prime Minister and at first kept Herbert in the Cabinet. But when Palmerston failed to make the House of Commons drop its plan to conduct the public enquiry, Sidney Herbert resigned because it was bound to discredit him in his previous involvement as Secretary at War. Florence Nightingale had lost an important supporter

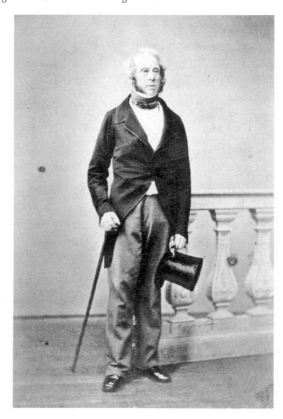

Lord Palmerston in the 1860s.

in the government, but she had gained Lord Palmerston who was even more supportive in his unobtrusive way.

The House of Commons Committee began to listen to evidence on 5 March, and its report, known as the Sebastopol Report, shows that Florence Nightingale's hospitals at Scutari came in for a good deal of criticism because of the chaotic supply arrangements there. Bandages, brushes and mops, kitchen utensils, beds and clothing all seemed to be in short supply despite the millions of pounds' worth of goods sent out from England. But the report praised Nightingale for rectifying the shortages using her own financial resources and those of *The Times*.

On the day that the Sebastopol Committee began to hear evidence in London, Nightingale was visited at Scutari by the ghost of Athena, an owl that she had once kept as a pet. She wrote to her family the next day describing the apparition:

Dearest people,
I saw Athena last night. She came to see me. I was walking home late from the General Hospital round the cliff, my favorite way, and looking, I really believe for the first time, at the view – the sea glassy calm

and of the purest sapphire blue, one solitary bright star rising above
Constantinople, our whole fleet standing with sails idly spread to catch
the breeze which was none, the domes and minarets of Constantinople
sharply standing out against the bright gold of the sunset, the transparent
opal of the distant hills (a colour one never sees but in the East) which
stretch below Olympus always snowy and on the other side the Sea of
Marmara, when Athena came along the cliff quite to my feet, rose upon
her tiptoes, bowed several times, made her long melancholy cry, and fled
away . . .

In London, the new government did not believe that a committee sitting
in the House of Commons could solve problems 3,000 miles away on
the Black Sea. Palmerston had his own ideas about what was wrong at
Scutari and in the Crimea and immediately on becoming Prime Minister

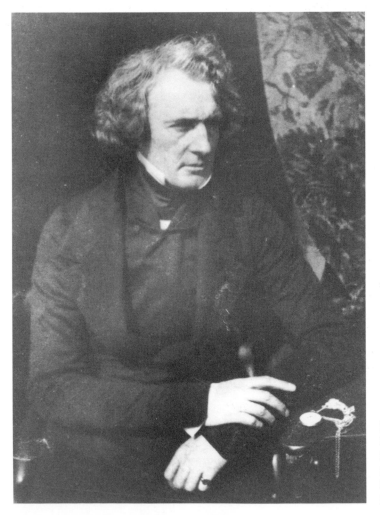

Sir John
McNeill
in 1845.
(© National
Portrait Gallery,
London)

despatched five men to investigate and take action on the spot, highly qualified civilians whom he could trust. The splendid British fleet becalmed in front of Stamboul that evening, on which Nightingale stood gazing down while she listened to a ghostly owl at her feet, included a vessel containing Palmerston's five commissioners, who disembarked the next day at Scutari. Their mission in the East was to save the British Army – the second British army to be sent there. The first army had already been lost.

The most eminent of these five commissioners was a man whose career brought to life to an almost unbelievable extent Nightingale's fantasies of philanthropic work accompanied by 'stirring events and romantic dangers'. He was Sir John McNeill, a sixty-year-old former diplomat who had been a key player in the 'Great Game' which pitted Britain against Russia in the struggle for control of central Asia. Although now retired from diplomacy, he was still active in the geopolitical arena and was publicly recognised at the time as bearing some responsibility for Britain's entry into the current war against Russia. He was famous both for this and for his private humanitarian efforts which had prevented the potato blight from causing mass famine in his native Scotland. Palmerston had chosen McNeill carefully for a most delicate task: he was deliberately to provoke a constitutional crisis in Britain in order to bring what at that time was still called the Queen's Army under the control of the House of Commons.

McNeill's enormous prestige, his powerful physique and still youthful looks, his record as a benefactor of the poor, and his insight into the most sensitive political affairs mesmerised Nightingale. She had cooled somewhat towards Sidney Herbert, her previous idol, as a result of his having broken his promise not to send out more nurses without her express consent. She was not particularly outraged by Herbert's fall from grace at home – the shortcomings of his government had been too widely publicised. And the waning of her high admiration for the surgeon MacGrigor coincided with McNeill's arrival. If ever there was an eminent man who merited the phrase *sui generis* – in a class of his own – it was McNeill. His life was so colourful that his private papers are still closely guarded, and anything published from them must be authorised by his descendents. A reliance on what is already publicly known seems to be the safer course, and reveals much.

Palmerston's decision to send McNeill to intervene in army matters was to bring him into conflict with Queen Victoria, not for the first time in his long career. Eventually Florence Nightingale was to become a pawn in this conflict, as Palmerston used her to thwart the Queen's attempts to claim control over the army for herself and her husband. The control of England's army had been a bone of contention since the reign of Charles I. During the Crimean War, disputes were common over whether the Commander-in-Chief in London's Horse Guards Parade took orders from the Queen herself or from her Ministers. In the Duke of Wellington's time, the question had never really arisen. Because of the enormous prestige he carried as the victor of Waterloo, as Commander-in-Chief, Wellington had almost absolute power over the army. But when he died in 1852 the old problems came to the surface and Queen Victoria, Prince Albert, and their allies tried to turn back the constitutional clock and re-establish royal control.

At the beginning of the war, Victoria had been on the throne for seventeen years but was still only thirty-five years old – one year older than Florence Nightingale. In her youth, Victoria was a very unpopular monarch due to her continental ancestry, her choice of a foreign husband, and the widely reported unfair treatment of one of her ladies-in-waiting who died after Victoria and her doctors diagnosed a tumour as an illicit pregnancy. After he became Prime Minister in 1855, Palmerston wanted to confine her interest to the more ceremonial aspects of military affairs. For example, he allowed her to change the design of the Victoria Cross. She threw out many cheap-looking and inferior designs proposed by civil servants for this 'all ranks' bravery medal and rejected their suggested motto *For the brave* because it implied that anyone who didn't have it wasn't brave. That is why this most coveted and rare decoration, of all times and all countries, bears Victoria's own words: *For Valour.*

Both Queen Victoria and her husband were military enthusiasts who followed army affairs closely and felt they had the right to control the army as well as design its medals. The Army High Command, which had been severely criticised in parliament, had everything to gain by encouraging this Royal interest and persuading the Queen that ancient, unwritten, constitutional principles required her to exert her nominal authority as head of the army and keep the House of Commons out of it. Palmerston was of the opposite view, which is why the Queen had tried everything possible to avoid making him Prime Minister after the previous government fell. While she cast forlornly around for other candidates she had left the country without a government for several days, at war against the biggest empire in the world, and with its army abandoned in an arctic hell. When she finally got the message that nobody would join a government unless her hated Palmerston was their leader, the stage was set for an epic confrontation that had been long in the making. Palmerston's first government appointment had been as Secretary of State at War nearly half a century before, and as long ago as 1812 he had argued that parliament and ministers could issue orders to the army independent of the Sovereign. Queen Victoria had engineered his dismissal as Foreign Secretary three years before for applying the same principle: he had sent a message to a foreign ruler without first clearing it with her.

Now, for Palmerston, it was payback time. His first act as Prime Minister was to send his civilian commissioners to the Crimea, and in McNeill's case he hid the true nature of the mission from the Queen and the army. He told them McNeill would investigate why the Commissariat, a civilian department of the Treasury, was failing to supply the army adequately; in reality McNeill was sent to investigate why the army was failing to inform the Commissariat of what was needed and failing to ask what they had in store. Junior officers had been resigning in droves since the landings in the Crimea; more than 10 per cent of them had gone home during the winter never to return, and they took home horrifying tales of the cruelty and indifference of senior officers towards their troops. One army captain even entitled his account *The Murder of a Regiment*. The best and most experienced Divisional Commander, General Sir George de Lacy Evans,

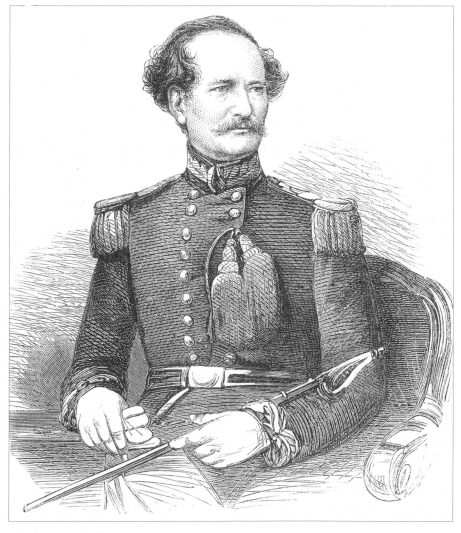

Sir Alexander Tulloch.

had quit the Crimea in disgust after the Commander-in-Chief rejected his plea to let the army spend the winter nearer to its supply port of Balaclava. McNeill had been well briefed on the details brought back to England by these critics, and later the army was to complain that his damning report had been written before he left England.

McNeill spent only a few days at Scutari *en route* to the Crimea, but during that time he wrote to British Consuls in friendly provinces surrounding the Black Sea asking them to send additional supplies to the Crimea. This far exceeded his instructions but he had spent too long as Palmerston's Minister Plenipotentiary and Envoy Extraordinary in Persia, a position carrying the power to wage war, to worry about his actions being questioned at home. He also met Nightingale and was at least as impressed with her as she was with him. In fact he was so impressed that his fellow commissioner Colonel Tulloch later refused to sign their joint report until McNeill removed a section which, according to Tulloch, betrayed his 'feelings' for her. Tulloch was an excitable and indiscreet man, though very able and protective of the troops, and his admonition to McNeill was more likely to have been a reaction to the obvious Nightingale-McNeill chemistry than to anything in McNeill's draft report. It was not the only source of friction between them. But before they left Scutari for the Crimea both Supplies Commissioners weighed in on the side of Nightingale and her ally MacGrigor in a row with their superiors over the unauthorised expenditure of hospital equipment.

Besides the Supplies Commission of McNeill and Tulloch, Palmerston had sent a Sanitary Commission to Scutari and the Crimea with more explicit instructions to clean up the camps and hospitals. It consisted of two doctors, Sutherland and Gavin, an engineer, Rawlinson, and a number of grandly titled Inspectors of Nuisances from Liverpool. They started literally at the bottom of the top, in the lavatory of the lazy aristocratic Commandant at Scutari. The Cabinet in London was gratified to receive a 'Report by Mr James Wilson, Inspector of Nuisances at Scutari Hospitals', which observed that 'The water-closet attached to Lord William Paulet's quarters being in an offensive state, I cleansed it myself.' Paulet was replaced and sent to the front.

Sutherland and his colleagues buried the dead animals that littered the site, paved and drained the yard outside the buildings, cleaned out the aqueduct and built a system to flush water through the sewers that ran under the building. They painted the internal walls with disinfectant and made openings in the roof of the building at strategic places to ensure ventilation.

Nightingale's own sanitary exertions had focused on the personal cleanliness of the patients; she had tried to wash and de-louse them and give them clean clothes. The nearest she got to environmental improvements had been an attempt to clean the floors. She had ordered quantities of mops, scrubbing brushes, and bottles of disinfectant. But the wooden floors of the wards were so rotten that they were hard to clean, and the broken and porous tiled floors in the corridors were hard to get at because of the densely packed straw mattresses on which the soldiers lay. Nightingale's main area of reform had been in disentangling hospital supplies from a mass of red tape, which is why she found a kindred spirit in McNeill, the Supplies Commissioner.

After McNeill and the other commissioners left for the Crimea, spring came to the Bosphorus. The nightingales sang in the old Turkish cemetery behind the hospital, and the Judas-trees put out their myriad pink flowers. The death rate in the hospitals seemed to abate and the number of sick sent down from the front declined as the Russian winter passed and the supplies to keep the soldiers healthy began to arrive in the camp. A steam tug appeared at Scutari from England, easing the task of getting sick soldiers ashore from the transports.

It was soon after the commissioners left that MacGrigor reported that Miss Nightingale wanted to go to the Crimea herself, a trip which would have qualified MacGrigor for a medal as soon as he stepped off the ship in Balaclava. But Nightingale did not need his company when she set off for the Crimea at the beginning of May 'to overhaul the Regimental Hospitals' as she put it. The Commander-in-Chief Lord Raglan had announced his intention of keeping the sick and wounded in the Crimea as much as possible. This reduced the workload at Scutari, and beds and other basic necessities had by now arrived and Nightingale's administrative duties there had become more manageable. For the remaining twelve months of the war, the extent of her authority in the Crimea was to remain a source of contention and much of her energy was devoted to defending it against opposition from rebellious nurses and jealous doctors. It would not be until the closing days of the war that the government would issue a General Order confirming that she was in charge of the nurses in the Crimea and rebuking those who had questioned her authority. Meanwhile, the question grew in importance as fewer patients came to the Bosphorus and more were hospitalised in the Crimea, and Nightingale made several trips from Scutari to the front to try to establish her authority.

When she went to the Crimea for the first time in May 1855, there were eight female nursing staff already there in the party that had left with Mrs Davis as described earlier. In April, the War Office had appointed Nightingale 'Almoner of the free gifts in all the British hospitals in the Crimean war zone' and this gave her an official capacity in which to visit the hospitals there even if her authority as Superintendent of Nurses was still disputed. She set sail for Balaclava in the Crimea on 5 May, 'having been at Scutari this day six months and, in sympathy with God, fulfilling the purpose I came into this world for'.

According to the rebellious Mrs Davis, during this visit to Balaclava Nightingale arranged a meeting with Dr John Hall, the army's Principal Medical Officer. Hall had recently become notorious for instructing surgeons not to use anaesthetics during amputations, and had been well known before that for his involvement in the case of a soldier who had died after being given 150 lashes. Hall had examined the soldier and had been present at his death; he gave his opinion at the inquest that the death was a consequence of a change in the weather rather than the flogging. He felt it necessary to observe to the coroner that he had seen many men flogged and had never heard from any of them such complaints as those made by the deceased. Possibly influenced by this gratuitous observation, the civilian coroner ignored Hall's opinion and found that the army had flogged the man to death. Hall was obviously not a man who owed his elevated position in the army to his defence of the rights of the common soldier.

Nightingale should logically have treated Hall as her superior, but Hall deliberately stayed clear of Scutari after she arrived, and she avoided recognising his authority over her or any female nurses. As the war continued, clashes between them became more and more frequent as they competed for control of groups of nurses at various locations. During her first visit to the Crimea, Nightingale presented Hall and his colleagues with a scheme for introducing a new system of hospital supplies management in the Crimea but they refused to accept it. Nightingale's intrusion into non-nursing matters understandably increased Hall's hostility. No doubt Sir John McNeill had a hand in the design of her proposed system for issuing supplies; he had been in the Crimea for two months interviewing army suspects who thought they were giving him evidence against the civilian Commissariat. Nightingale relied on him for moral support in this disputed territory.

Nightingale's letters home show that McNeill took her into his confidence about his enquiries, and the details distressed her. He told her that throughout the arctic winter the soldiers had nothing hot to drink unless they could grind up and roast raw green coffee beans; there was a huge quantity of tea in the army's stores but there was nothing in the ancient rule book about issuing tea to soldiers. And the rule book did not require the army to supply the men with cooking fuel either; they had to obtain it themselves and there was none, unless they could claw a few roots out of the frozen ground. The friendly provinces around the Black Sea were wooded down to the shore, he said, and the Navy was on hand to fetch charcoal, but that was irrelevant to the Army High Command if the rule book didn't say anything about issuing fuel. He told her that the men could not eat the beef and pork preserved in salt, or the hard biscuit, because their gums were lacerated with scurvy, while cases of lime juice lay unopened in the army's stores. While the stipulated rations of salt meat were hauled up to the camp day after day and then dumped because the men could not eat it, the Commissary General said that he had no capacity left over for transporting the rice which was in store and would have cured the scurvy. They craved soft bread beyond all; the stores were full of flour, but no orders were given to build ovens like the French had done, and the men were worked too hard to do it themselves. They spent five nights out of seven sitting out in shallow ditches guarding against a surprise attack by the besieged Russians, often for 36 hours at a stretch. At the end of each shift, some were found dead of exposure or with their bare feet frozen to the ground. The army had deprived them of their knapsacks on their march along the coast, and all their personal belongings and spare clothing. The knapsacks had been stored somewhere but nobody knew where and that's why her patients were arriving in rags.

All this Nightingale listened to with mounting dismay and McNeill went remorselessly on, talking to a soft-hearted pillar of the English gentry as much as to a Superintendent of Nursing. This is what he planned to expose in parliament, he told her. About the raw recruits, shipped out from England without training, left alone on the shore with no shelter and nobody to guide them to camp, sickening and dying immediately. About Lord Raglan having the effrontery to ask the Minister of War to kindly send out only recruits who could survive sleeping out in the open in winter. About how Raglan had given orders to abandon the supply port of Balaclava after having failed to resist the capture of the only road from it to the camp. About how he had countermanded the order without telling the ships that had been ordered out of the port and told to anchor against a lee shore, so that when the hurricane came dozens of them were wrecked with the loss of thousands of lives and millions in stores.

Scandalised, Nightingale wrote to her family passing on some of McNeill's confidential criticisms of the army and singling him out for praise: 'Sir John McNeill is the man I like the best of all who has come out. He has dragged the Commissary General out of the mud. He has done wonders. Everybody now has their fresh meat three times a week, their fresh bread from Constantinople about as often.' Then she wrote: 'Sir John McNeill whom you must not quote, told me that it was . . .' Her letter to her family breaks off here and we don't know for sure what the next secret was going to be, but a good guess is that it was at this point that he told her why the soldiers sent to her hospital in the winter could not have been cured. They had been starved to death, he said, nothing could have been done to save them. He had discovered that the men had been on half rations, quarter rations, or no rations at all for days on end.

McNeill had trained as a doctor, so his diagnosis carried weight with Nightingale. He was also one of the few people around with previous first-hand experience of a siege like the one the British were conducting here. In 1837 he had persuaded the Persians to end their siege of Herat in Afghanistan, which they were conducting at the suggestion of the Russians who wanted to destabilise Afghanistan and threaten India. McNeill predicted that the siege would fail because of starvation among the attackers, not the defenders, although his more powerful argument was propounded in his suspension of diplomatic relations with Persia and summoning of gunboats from Britain to the Gulf. His more recent experience of the effects of starvation had come from an official tour of the Highlands and Islands, in his capacity as Chairman of the Scottish equivalent of the Poor Law Board, at a time when the area was suffering from potato crop failure. The actions he took avoided the mass starvation that occurred in Ireland.

Nightingale heard all about McNeill's extraordinary career, both from the man himself and from awed gossip in the camp. Nothing could more closely resemble the life of 'stirring events and romantic dangers' that she had fantasised about sharing with a man. At the age of nineteen, McNeill had gone to India with his bride of sixteen and their baby daughter to seek his fortune with the East India Company as an Assistant Surgeon. India had killed his young wife within two years; he had sent the child home and gone on active service with the Company's army, battling and intriguing against the country's bandits. He survived long enough to become a skilled physician and negotiator, and the Company sent him to be medical officer to the British Mission (and to the Shah's household) in Persia when he was only twenty-five. His skill at 'harem diplomacy' led to his promotion to Minister Plenipotentiary, even higher than Ambassador. He was Palmerston's most trusted envoy during his long reign as Foreign Secretary, which was so foolishly curtailed by Victoria and her boot-licking Prime Minister.

McNeill, having got Nightingale's attention with his heartbreaking and highly confidential account of the aristocracy's mistreatment of the British common soldier during the terrible winter above Sebastopol, told her about his adventures in Persia opposing the Russians and the grudge the Tsar bore him. It wasn't just that McNeill was the author of books calling on Britain and France to attack Russia, writing just before the joint declaration of war: 'Let us hope that our tardiness to accept the combat is but an indication that we foresee its magnitude; and that the two great Western Powers warned as it were by a mighty voice from the tomb against a little war [a reference to a supposed quotation from the late Duke of Wellington] are prepared, if negotiation has failed, at once to put forth all their strength – to hit hard – and to strike home.' This had only been a warning to Russia, written for his friend Palmerston who was unable to deliver the warning in person after Victoria had kicked him out of the Foreign Office. Russia's grudge against McNeill went back a long way further than that. It is easy to imagine him holding Nightingale spellbound with his version of Griboyedov's murder, recounting it in a flimsy shack on the edge of the Crimean plain while Russian Cossack horsemen prowled close by searching for unwary strays from the British camp. Perhaps Nightingale and McNeill were at a makeshift dinner with a group of officers when one of them asked McNeill what really happened in Teheran in 1829. If so we can imagine McNeill not talking to Nightingale directly, but being aware of her eyes fixed on him as wide as saucers.

Alexander Griboyedov, still today one of Russia's best-known playwrights, had been appointed Russian Ambassador to Teheran in 1828. Under the terms of the latest treaty between Persia and Russia, Persia had agreed to return slaves whom they had abducted from Russian territory. According to McNeill, Griboyedov had identified some of these slaves and had taken three Persian girls hostage when their owners failed to deliver the slaves to his Embassy. The Persian girls escaped onto the roof and called out to passers-by that they had been sexually molested, whereupon an armed mob descended on the Embassy and murdered almost everyone in it, including Ambassador Griboyedov. Rumours circulated in Russian circles at the time that the Shah had organised the mob, aided and abetted by McNeill who had become his close confidant and personal physician after successfully treating his favourite wife and her son, and who had been opposing Russia's expansionist intrigues in Persia for years.

There is no possibility that McNeill had anything to do with Griboyedov's murder, although during the Cold War, Soviet historians dusted off the story and pretended to believe it. But at Sebastopol in 1855, the thought that McNeill was risking capture by the Russians who believed him guilty of such a heinous crime added even more romance to his name. For Nightingale his life story was a chat-up line that could not fail, given her wish to serve a brave, humane, and masculine leader. For the next two years, as McNeill became increasingly embroiled in the constitutional crisis that he and Palmerston had engineered, Nightingale was McNeill's most ardent supporter, and when she returned home she placed herself directly under his orders for the final act of the struggle. Palmerston would eventually win his fight for control of the Army, of Foreign Policy, and of everything else, and Nightingale was to be the instrument with which he and McNeill finally taught Victoria to be a constitutional Queen.

Did McNeill and Nightingale have a battlefield romance? Yes, in the sense of a mutual infatuation: letters between them and remarks by their colleagues show a relationship going beyond friendship, as we shall see. It may have been a physical relationship; so little is known nowadays about

Victorian sexual practices that we cannot be certain. During the war they were together a week at Scutari, then a month in the Crimea during part of which time she was intermittently ill, then perhaps a week at Scutari before he returned to England. It is commonly believed that Victorians could not enjoy extramarital sex because of fear of pregnancy and disease, but there is plenty of evidence that satisfactory non-penetrative sex was safely practiced and Nightingale's 'dreaming' seems to show that she was erotically charged. They were often alone together discussing their respective secret missions and her illness provided another point of confidential discussion. It must be borne in mind that he was a doctor, one who had practiced his craft in the harem.

At sixty, McNeill was twenty-five years older than Nightingale, but this was in an age when women were often married to much older men, partly as a result of high mortality in childbirth. According to his granddaughter, McNeill was known as 'the handsomest man in Edinburgh'; he wore his hair unconventionally long as shown in the photographs of him in the National Portrait Gallery and in the marble bust which John Steel made at about the time of the Crimean War. He was the same age as her father, that beloved but (according to Nightingale) ineffectual man who had never 'carried anything out'. McNeill could not be accused of having that particular flaw. He had married again after his first wife died, but his second wife had refused to follow him abroad for the last six years of his Persian adventures after four of their five children had died young – a son and two daughters in Persia and another daughter in Scotland while her parents were abroad. Naturally enough, Lady McNeill did not share her husband's insatiable love of adventure and wanted to protect their only surviving child.

On her thirty-fifth birthday, Nightingale fell ill in the Crimea and was in bed with fever for about ten days, during which time McNeill visited her bedside. We know this from Charles Bracebridge, the husband of the close friend of Nightingale who had accompanied her to the Crimea and who had earlier noted Nightingale's need to meet her male colleagues unchaperoned. Nightingale disliked Bracebridge and only tolerated him because of his wife; it was he who had made the careless remark that led to Sidney Herbert sending out more nurses against Nightingale's wishes, and she could not forgive him. Bracebridge, writing to Nightingale's family, shows that the camp was well aware of McNeill's reputation: 'I met Sir John McNeill there [at the hospital where Mrs Roberts, her housekeeper, was caring for Nightingale]. He was questioning Mrs. Roberts about her with as much interest as he ever did the Shah's ministers.' Bracebridge returned to his preoccupation with McNeill in another letter: 'Sir John McNeill has taken a great fancy for Flo and goes up most evenings to enquire, & sometimes sees her.' This strong language for Victorian times about a married man would make Nightingale's family uneasy, especially in the light of her earlier fulsome praise of McNeill. Bracebridge was telling tales out of jealousy.

While recovering from her illness, Nightingale wrote McNeill a peculiar letter which has defied interpretation until now and has always been described as the product of delirium during her fever. Surprisingly, it is written in her most impeccable copperplate script. It is partly in code, and if her prudish relatives had understood it they would have destroyed it after her death. 'Dear Sir John,' she wrote, 'I can hardly tell what brings me to you. Last week a Persian adventurer appeared to me like a phantom, showed me papers by which Mr Bracebridge seemed to have drawn upon me for £300,000. I sent for him. He [Bracebridge] said very little, neither denied nor assented but said no one would ever believe that I had seen the papers there for the first time. This is all, dear Sir John, that I have to say. Have you any advice to give? I come to you because you have shewn me much kindness. Dear Sir John, Yours truly, Florence Nightingale.'

Any letter is a collaborative venture between sender and recipient, and the key to decoding this one is to put yourself in McNeill's place and realise that he would know instantly that he must be the 'Persian adventurer' who appeared in her dream. Probably it was a term he had used to her to downplay his extraordinary career. Far from being the most obscure part of the letter, the Persian adventurer sequence is the most lucid if read correctly. The rest resembles the feelings we have in awaking from a vivid dream – we realise with one part of the mind that the events didn't happen, but nevertheless they still seem 'real' and worrying.

Regardless of whether any of the other events described in Nightingale's letter actually happened, and how delirious she was when she wrote it, it is clear that Nightingale told Sir John that she had dreamed of his coming to her rescue. Furthermore, she felt guilty enough about the inappropriate feelings that this revealed to write in code – a code enigmatic enough to escape the censors after her death. This shows that McNeill's 'great fancy' was mutual.

One reason that attracted her to McNeill was the reassurance he gave that there was nothing she could have done to save the men who died in such large numbers in her hospital in the winter. His first report, written while he was still in the Crimea, focussed almost entirely on bad diet as the reason for the 'expenditure of men' as he called it: 'the same unvarying diet of salt meat and biscuit, without a sufficient supply of vegetables, produced scurvy, which rendered more fatal almost every other disease by which the men were attacked in December and January.' This was reassuring because since August the previous year there had been complaints that the Scutari Barrack Hospital building was filthy to the point of endangering the health of its inmates. The medical hierarchy had insisted that nothing was wrong, the Principal Medical Officer Dr Hall writing in his report on the hospital the previous October 'the sick and wounded are all doing as well as could possibly be expected . . . our difficulties have been in great measure surmounted, and in a short time, I flatter myself, we shall have a hospital establishment that will bear a comparison with any other one of the same magnitude formed under similar disadvantages, or indeed I may almost venture to say, under any circumstances.' Close examination shows a few carefully placed weasel words here, such as the 'almost' that can pass unnoticed on the first reading.

Despite Hall's optimism, there must still have been speculation in London that conditions at Scutari were partly responsible for the high death rate there during the first winter, because Nightingale wrote to the new Minister of War denying this possibility. She blamed the men's deaths on their moribund state when they arrived, as per McNeill's diagnosis: 'The physically deteriorating effect of the Scutari air has been much discussed, but it may be doubted. The men sent down to Scutari in the winter died because they were not sent down till half dead – the men sent down now live and recover because they are sent in time.'

While in the Crimea, Nightingale also met Lord Raglan, the Commander-in-Chief. She wrote to her father proudly that she had upheld the honour of the family like a son: 'Lord Raglan asked me if my father liked me coming out to the East. I said with pride that my father is not as other men are. He thinks that daughters should serve their country as well as sons. He brought me up to think so; he has no sons, and therefore he has sacrificed me to my country, and told me to come home with my shield or upon it. He thinks that God sent women, as well as men, into the world to be something more than "happy", "attentive" and "amusing". My father's religious and social ethics make us strive to be the pioneers of the human race, and let "happiness" and "amusement" take care of themselves.'

When she was convalescing from her illness, Nightingale was given the use of a private yacht to carry her back to Scutari. It was owned by Lord Ward, an eccentric coal millionaire who had come out to the Crimea as a tourist bringing gifts for the troops. Bracebridge wrote: 'We hope to go down to Scutari with Sir John McNeill & perhaps come back here again if she be well enough.' It is not known whether McNeill did travel on Lord Ward's yacht, but he left the Crimea and arrived at Scutari on the same dates, and even if he did not accompany her the thought, according to Bracebridge, was there.

She had to visit the Crimea again four months later. It was after the hospital at Kulali, 5 miles from Scutari, closed down in October 1855. The nurses there were Irish sisters headed by one of Nightingale's rivals: they had been in the second party sent out by Sidney Herbert for which Nightingale had refused to accept responsibility. Now her opponent Dr

John Hall invited them to take up residence in the Crimea; to preserve her authority over them, Nightingale had to take them there. This visit led to further wrangling between Nightingale and Hall and between nurses aligned with each camp. Things developed to such a state that the Minister of War asked his confidential aide-de-camp, Colonel Lefroy, to investigate Nightingale's quarrels with the Hall faction.

A later confidential task entrusted to Lefroy was to help to persuade Nightingale to fight for reform after the war, a decision that she eventually took as a result of a direct appeal from Lord Palmerston. As a reward for his many discreet services, Lefroy was later granted his wish to be allowed to set up an army educational corps to improve the common soldier. He seems to have been one of the many advanced thinkers who associated themselves with the army because it allowed them to experiment with their social theories. His interests were wide-ranging: he had spent many months in the wilderness of northern Canada, carrying out important studies of the earth's magnetic field, but his main passion apart from running schools for soldiers was cataloguing obsolete cannons.

Not surprisingly in view of his interest in educating the common soldier, Lefroy and Nightingale got on very well at their first meeting and Lefroy reported to his superiors that she was in the right and Hall was in the wrong. He convinced the Cabinet to clarify and extend Nightingale's responsibilities. But when Nightingale demanded that Sidney Herbert make her disputes with Hall the subject of a parliamentary enquiry, the Cabinet decided to give her some advice on public relations. Sidney Herbert, who had originally sent Nightingale to the East, was no longer a Minister, but Nightingale continued to use him as her intermediary with the government. The government in turn used Herbert as her 'handler'. It may have been at the Cabinet's suggestion that Herbert wrote her a masterly letter early in 1856 telling her that she had everything to lose and nothing to gain by airing her quarrels in public.

Herbert told her that it would not be in her interest to present to parliament her strongly worded denunciations of her rivals. 'The reader seeing the vehemence of your language would at once say. "This is written under great irritation and I must take its statements with suspicion," and he chooses for himself what to put aside as the result of anger and perhaps puts aside just what you most rely on in your statement.' He advised her to calm down and not attribute base motives to her rivals in her dispatches, in case they should become public. He compared the 'irritation and vehemence' of her written reports with the 'sobriety of tone' and calm marshalling of facts in McNeill's report on the supply blunders of the army, which had just been published in London. Herbert told her that McNeill had reported only objective facts, leaving the reader to imagine to himself what base motives must lie behind them: 'The public like to have something left to their own imaginations and are much pleased with their own sagacity when they have found out what was too obvious to be missed. It is always wise too in a public document to understate your case. If on examination your case proves stronger than you stated it to be, you reap the whole advantage. If however, any part, however slight, is shaken, the credit of the whole is shaken with it.'

Herbert's letter infuriated Nightingale. She fired back a response accusing Herbert of always ducking a quarrel and trying to smooth things over as he had done in parliament as Minister at War when he had brushed aside complaints about the mistreatment of the troops. If she was 'quarrelling', she asked, does that mean that Joan of Arc was 'quarrelling' with the English? She accused Herbert of lazing beside the fire while the Principal Medical Officer in the Crimea was deliberately withholding rations to starve her, and she claimed that McNeill's report would have achieved nothing on its own – it had been his readiness to 'put his hand to the plough' out here that had saved the army. It is true that the powerful army lobby was now comprehensively denouncing McNeill's report while the government seemed reluctant to defend it, so its effectiveness was in doubt. One of the two men most severely criticised in it was Dr John Hall, Nightingale's principal opponent, but he was knighted only three weeks after its publication. It seemed likely that McNeill's report was being buried.

Not all of Nightingale's time was spent quarrelling, and the large amount of correspondence on the subject is misleading. It is worth noting that she knew that the correspondence does not always show her in a good light, but it was she who ensured that it would be preserved for posterity as a history lesson. Despite the fireworks, she put more effort into improving the lot of the common soldier than in fighting Hall. Her belief in the common soldier's innate perfectibility was an intellectual position arising from Unitarian influences. She wrote to the Dean of Hereford asking him to send out (and bill her father for) emphatically not bibles, but paper, pens, and ink, encyclopaedias, and diagrams of natural history and the stratification of the earth, for lectures. As for the officers, they should study trigonometry. Like so many others at that time, she was coming to see the army as a proving ground for her social theories.

Lord William Paulet (he of the remarkably dirty lavatory) had accused Nightingale of 'spoiling those brutes' – pointing contemptuously to the soldiers who were carried back insensible from the Greek drinking dens and frequently died without regaining consciousness. The Cabinet had requested Paulet to use his considerable powers to put a stop to such waste of life. Paulet limited himself to preventing the sale of spirits in the hospital itself. Nightingale's plan was to give the soldiers some other way to spend their time and their pay. Taken in isolation, her letters may give the impression that laundries, kitchens, money order offices, reading rooms, and lectures would never have appeared if she had not organised them. However, independent evidence that her role was very important comes from the reaction to her initiative to reduce drunkenness.

Nightingale wrote to Queen Victoria that drunkenness in the army would be reduced if it were made easier for soldiers to send home their pay by opening Post Office branches where they could buy and send home postal orders in private. When her letter was read to Palmerston's Cabinet, all present complemented it except the Minister of War who said it showed that Nightingale 'knew nothing of the British soldier'. The Generals in the Crimea refused to countenance her idea on principle, representing as it did civilian interference. Nightingale sweetly backed down, but reminded the Generals that as there was now a large corps of well-paid and somewhat riotous civilian navvies in the Crimea, it would be desirable to open Post Office branches for civilians. This the army could not object to; the soldiers flocked to them, the amount of money sent home made a significant impact on the domestic economy, and the problem of chronic drunkenness ceased. When the Commander-in-Chief complained, the Minister of War sympathised with him and blamed it all on agitation by Nightingale: 'The great cry now, and Miss Nightingale inflames it, is that the men have no means to remit their money home. This is not true. The soldier may remit his money through the Paymaster, with no trouble at all. We have now offered the Post Office to them, but I am sure it will do no good. The soldier is not a remitting animal.' Being a close ally of Palmerston's, he almost certainly said this just to pretend to the Army High Command that they had a supporter in the Cabinet. But whether he was sincere or just putting on a front for the Generals, his comments illustrate the effectiveness of Nightingale's high-level interference and the obstacles that she skilfully overcame.

She was proud of her record, and scornful of her detractors, as she showed when asking her sister Parthenope to lobby the government for a monument to honour the Scutari dead: 'Five thousand and odd brave hearts sleep here. We have endured in brave Grecian silence. We have folded our mantles about our faces and died in silence without complaining. And for myself, I have done my duty. I have identified my fate with that of the heroic dead, and whatever lies these officials, these sordid exploiters of human misery, spread about us, there is a right and a God to fight for and our fight has been worth fighting. I do not complain. It has been a great cause.' All Britain was proud of her, too. Her illness at Balaclava had caused consternation in the newspapers at home, and the news of her recovery had led to national rejoicing. The public was impressed when after her convalescence at Scutari she decided not to return home but to remain at her post. Sidney Herbert decided to exploit the national wave of enthusiasm and sympathy to launch a national appeal for funds to support her – and his – scheme to improve the standard of female nursing in civilian hospitals. Herbert and the other politicians were pleased to be able to point to one good thing that had come out of a war that was otherwise a catalogue of disasters.

Before the war, Nightingale had resigned from her first hospital position so that she could seek another where she could train nurses. While she was in the East, a doctor whom she knew had written to her to suggest that she help him to establish a school for nurses in one of London's teaching hospitals. Herbert set up a committee to raise money for the project. The exact wording of the committee's resolution for raising money is important because of the obligation that it placed on Florence Nightingale 'on her return to England, to establish a permanent institution for the training of nurses and to arrange for their proper instruction and employment *in hospitals*'. The last two words were to cause her trouble later when she wanted to divert some of the funds to training nurses to work outside hospitals. At a public meeting in London at the end of November 1855, Herbert launched a national appeal for subscriptions to the 'Nightingale Fund'. The meeting was packed to suffocation and delirious in its praise of the faraway heroine. Herbert read out to the adoring crowd a letter from a soldier who had been in Nightingale's crowded hospital: 'What a comfort it was to see her pass. She would speak to one and nod and smile to many more, but she could not do it to all, you know. We lay there by hundreds; but we would kiss her shadow as it fell, and lay our heads on the pillow again, content.'

The appeal for subscriptions brought in a sum worth several million pounds in today's money, to fund the training of hospital nurses. Queen Victoria sent Nightingale an inscribed diamond brooch and an invitation to meet her when she returned to England. The soldier's letter which launched the Nightingale Fund also inspired a poem by Longfellow which immortalised the Nightingale legend:

> *Lo! In that hour of misery*
> *A lady with a lamp I see*
> *Pass through the glimmering gloom,*
> *And flit from room to room.*
> *And slow, as in a dream of bliss,*
> *The speechless sufferer turns to kiss Her shadow, as it falls.*

Nightingale's mother and sister were ecstatic with pride after the public meeting in London. Her mother wrote: 'It is very late, my child, but I cannot go to bed without telling you that your meeting has been a glorious one.' Her father was more reserved but could not conceal his 'Joy at the meeting which has honoured Flo with its absolute finding of "Well done".

I am not easily satisfied but all people seem to agree that there was there nothing wanting.'

After the bitter disagreements over her desire to take up nursing the approval of her family was far more important to Nightingale than public fame. 'If my name and having done what I could for God and mankind has given you pleasure that is real pleasure to me' she wrote in reply to her mother's description of Herbert's public meeting. 'My reputation has not been a boon to me in my work – but if you have been pleased, that is enough. I shall love my name now. Life is sweet after all.' She was now famous, and the evidence of her success in the hospitals, and that of McNeill on supplies at the front, was visible. The British Army in the East was in fine health. In five months during the first winter of the war, 10,000 British soldiers had died of sickness, but in the same five months during the second winter only 500 men died out of an army that was now swollen to twice the size. The improvement was not only due to a milder winter, for during that second winter the death rate in the French Army *increased* by 60 per cent. This was largely due to the failure of the French supply chain, because they had extended their lines to occupy a valley south of Sebastopol. In the first winter the French had all been within a short distance of their supply port at Kamiesch, while the British had been miles from Balaclava and had not yet built their railway.

In the spring of 1856, the War Office issued a General Order to the army, specifying once and for all that Nightingale's authority extended to all the hospitals, those in the Crimea as well as those on the Bosphorus. She immediately set sail for the Crimea and took possession of Balaclava General Hospital, where Dr (now Sir) John Hall the previous October had installed a party of nurses who preferred to be independent of Nightingale. The rival nurses now resigned and went home rather than work under her command.

The war officially ended on 30 March 1856 when the Treaty of Paris was signed. Britain and her allies had forced the Russians to evacuate the dockyards of Sebastopol, and destroyed the docks with great ceremony. It was not the victory that Palmerston had hoped for, and the totalitarian Russian Empire continued to grow even more than he had feared, from then until 1989.

Nightingale stayed on in the Crimea until every soldier had left. She began to have time to read the newspapers from England, and followed the debates in parliament, where the post-mortem on the war had already begun. Her hero Sir John McNeill's star seemed to be waning fast, as a public tribunal had rejected all of his criticisms. Army reform was to all appearances dead.

CHAPTER FOUR

Post-Mortem

She did not seem to be in a hurry to get home. After a subdued embarkation in the ravaged corner of Russia where the war had petered out many months before, Nightingale went ashore at Marseilles and made her way across France incognito, arriving in England on 6 August 1856. Perhaps she hung back because she was nervous about rejoining the world. In the two years since she had left home she had seen Constantinople ravaged by earthquake and fire, had held thousands of dying men in her arms, and had beaten the most powerful army in the world in a battle over the rights of common soldiers whether sick or healthy. What would she have in common with the people at home?

Postponing the reunion with her family, she first went to the Bermondsey Convent of the Sisters of Mercy where some of her wartime nursing companions had returned to work among London's destitute. They didn't have the problem of fitting back into family life because they had left it for good years ago. Founded by Catharine McAuley, an Irish orphan girl who inherited a fortune, the convent's mission was to minister to the sick poor in the filthiest slums. Being among them in England allowed Nightingale to feel that the real world still existed – the world of squalor and death and cruelty. The Bermondsey Sisters had been among her most loyal supporters in the hospitals in the Crimea and Turkey; she must have enjoyed a good gossip with them about the intrigues in the army and medical services in the East since the Sisters had come home three months earlier.

There was a more practical reason for her visit: the Sisters of Mercy had kept meticulous accounts and Nightingale needed these to help straighten out her own complicated financial situation arising from her expenditure in the East. She spent three weeks working on her accounts, first at the convent and then at the family home in Derbyshire, before turning to the question of her future career. She could now begin to openly plan a future in nursing administration. In this, she had the satisfaction of having won a great victory over her mother and sister. Public opinion, which before had been indisputably on their side, was now on hers: nursing had become a useful and respectable activity for women. She no longer had to seek her family's permission to follow her vocation.

She had no idea how she was going to make use of the fund that the public had subscribed in her name during the war for the training of nurses. She was now rather less interested in training nurses in a large teaching hospital than she had been before the war. She was more interested in hospital management: 'If I had a plan it would be simply to take the poorest and least organised hospital in London and putting myself there see what I could do not touching the Fund for years until experience had shown how the Fund might best be available.'

Nightingale described a slightly different plan when writing to her military friends, perhaps because she wanted to keep open as many options as possible. She told them that she wanted to work in army hospitals. Her letters reveal that she recognised the danger that this avenue might be closed if she allowed herself to be dragged into the controversy that still surrounded the loss of Britain's first army sent to the Crimea. She was convinced that the incompetence and heartlessness of the Army High Command had resulted in the deaths of thousands of common soldiers in the camps and hospitals during the winter of 1854. Two years had gone by since then and nobody had been reprimanded. On the contrary, the four officers most to blame had been promoted – even (or so it had been alleged in the House of Commons) after the government had in its hands the proof of their incompetence, namely McNeill's report.

The results of this incompetence had been visible in the stream of soldiers who were shipped to her hospital near Constantinople, dying from extreme malnutrition, exposure, and exhaustion. The men who had amazed the world with their courage at the Alma and at Balaclava had arrived scarcely alive, many having died in transit and many more dying soon after arriving at the hospital. Over 16,000 British soldiers had died of sickness, while fewer than 2,600 were killed in battle and 1,500 died of wounds. The hair-raising reports of treatment of the sick and wounded published in the newspapers had led to the fall of the government that had sent Nightingale to the East, but the Army High Command seemed to have emerged from the fuss unscathed. The public now seemed to have lost interest in McNeill's accusations that senior officers had made no attempt to feed and clothe the army properly, and had allowed the supplies already at their disposal to remain in store nearby while the troops died for lack of them.

Since the McNeill investigation, there had been a change in the political climate, and demand for army reform had decreased. Public dissatisfaction at the time of the disaster had forced a change of government, and death had replaced the Commander-in-Chief in the Crimea. The war was now over and the government appeared ready to let sleeping dogs lie. After the war's end, Nightingale was reluctant to make any public pronouncements at all. The use of female nurses in war was still controversial and she thought that if the women made themselves too visible it would play into the hands of those who were still opposed to the idea. She wrote:

> Now the war has ended and we return to England, the less we say about the last two years the better since not only we are the last appointed, the fewest, and the lowest in official rank of the Queen's war servants, but we are the first women who have been suffered in the war service. To return either sounding our own trumpet or, viler still, attacking the system under which, and because of which we worked, can only at once degrade ourselves, and justify, *pro tanto*, the common opinion that the vanity, the gossip and the insubordination of women (which none more despise than those who trade upon them) make them unfit and mischievous in the service, however materially useful they may be in it. Hospital nursing, to be anything other than a nuisance, must remain to the end of time a very humble as well as a very laborious drudgery. But, done aright for God and man, it is a noble work. Let us, please God our consciences bear us witness that we have tried to do our duty, hold fast our integrity nor let our hearts reproach us as long as we live.

She was only reluctantly willing to co-operate through the conventional channels with any official enquiry: 'I ought to show to the War Office that I am at hand to answer any questions,' Nightingale wrote while she was still in the Crimea, just before an official enquiry into McNeill's report had dismissed its criticisms of the army and exonerated the accused officers. This outcome surprised and shocked Nightingale, who passionately agreed with McNeill's report and had been following the enquiry from afar. The failure of McNeill's attempt to expose the cruel treatment of the common soldier must have heightened her sense of injustice, but it made her even less willing to give her opinion on army defects, even in confidence to her official superiors. She thought that she would be safer working for reform quietly behind the scenes. She feared that she might share the fate of McNeill and his assistant Colonel Tulloch, whose considerable reputations appeared to have been destroyed by Lord Palmerston's failure to support them after he had published their report.

Palmerston's government had sent two civilian-led commissions to the Crimea immediately upon taking office in February 1855. The report of Dr Sutherland's Sanitary Commission was still not published, but Sir John McNeill delivered his report while the war was still going on, and it was presented to parliament and published at the beginning of 1856, six months before Nightingale came home. It claimed that the incompetence or inaction of identified senior officers had caused the deaths of thousands of common soldiers through overwork, inadequate food and shelter, and scurvy. It said the disaster could have been prevented by the use of supplies that were either already in the army's stores or available in the near vicinity. The Crimean peninsula, as part of Russia, was enemy territory, but it was surrounded by Turkish provinces allied with Britain and plentifully stocked with the necessary supplies. They were distant only a few hours from the British camps by transport ships, of which the army had large numbers at its disposal.

Queen Victoria was furious that Palmerston's government had presented McNeill's criticism to the public for debate. Neither did she like the government's idea that the criticised officers should write out their defences for presentation to parliament. She recognised that this was an attempt by her Ministers to increase the involvement of the House of Commons in army affairs:

> A civil Commission is sent out by the Government to inquire into the conduct of the officers in command in the Crimea,' she wrote. 'It is quite evident that if matters are left so, and military officers of the Queen's Army are to be judged by a Committee of the House of Commons, the Command of the Army is at once transferred from the Crown to that Assembly. This result is quite inevitable if the Government appear as accusers, as they do by the report of their Commission, and then submit the accusations for Parliament to deal with without taking any steps of their own.

Palmerston believed that phrases like 'the Queen's Army', 'the Crown', and 'the Royal Prerogative' should now simply represent the additional power that Ministers had to act independently of parliament in certain areas when they judged it necessary. In his liberal view, there was no actual power vested in the Queen, though Ministers had to keep her informed and she might try to persuade them. The Queen herself, who had been instructed on the subject by the late Duke of Wellington, did not agree and neither did the Army High Command. Victoria was correct in her fear that if the government did not act on McNeill's report, but instead passed it to the House of Commons, it would be destroying the Crown Prerogative over the army. This government thought that it had the right to transfer command of the army from the Crown (i.e. Ministers acting undemocratically) to the House of Commons if the government so chose. Palmerston wanted parliament to debate any matter that required it to spend large amounts of money. In the past, parliament had been very parsimonious with the army because it did not have enough control over it, and this interfered with Palmerston's ambitious defence spending plans.

The government now dodged the issue by pretending that it had not authorised the investigation of army officers: 'The Commission of which Sir J. McNeill and Colonel Tulloch were members was sent out in February

1855 – their instructions bear date 19th of that month – to inquire into matters purely connected with Commissariat supplies to the Army.'

In specifying the date of the instructions as 19 February, the government was deliberately concealing the existence of supplementary instructions dated three days later which had given McNeill additional powers to investigate why supplies made available to the army by the Commissariat had not reached the soldiers. Both sets of instructions were printed at the front of the objectionable report, although the tiny supplementary instructions were printed separately high up on the back of a page where they were hard to spot. Queen Victoria and her husband had apparently not read the small print. In the Crimea, the commissioners must have shown their instructions without turning over the page.

When the Queen asked why the government did not strike out the parts of the report where the commissioners had exceeded their brief, she received the flimsy excuse that it would mean altering the evidence, which she would surely find unethical. She was not to know that the government *had* struck out some evidence: a table of sickness and mortality which could have hindered recruiting and would assume great importance later. Victoria suggested to Palmerston that the report should be investigated by an army Board of Generals, which would rule on the truthfulness of the allegations. The Queen assumed that the Board's enquiry would be held in secret, but this suggestion led to an uproar in parliament and the government had to declare that the proceedings would be open after all. The Queen was 'disappointed and annoyed' by this decision, but Palmerston pointed out that in arguing for a Board of Generals she had cited an 1808 precedent where a Board had been used, and in that case the proceedings had been open.

The government now conspicuously tried to avoid discussion of McNeill's report in parliament, the War Minister reluctantly admitting that he had commissioned it while giving the impression that he didn't agree with its findings. McNeill was surprised and offended by this refusal to publicly back his report, and was further offended when his request that his assistant Colonel Tulloch be promoted was rudely rebuffed. The Prime Minister, cornered in a House of Commons debate, was forced to give his own verdict on the report. To everybody's surprise Palmerston praised it and its authors to the skies. This annoyed McNeill even more when he read the account of the debate in the newspapers. He wrote to an acquaintance in the Cabinet demanding to know why Palmerston's Minister of War had given a completely different impression in public. Palmerston's praise had made McNeill think that the War Office was out of step with the government and was supporting the Queen and her Generals against Palmerston.

McNeill was determined to boycott the army's Board of Enquiry into his report, but worried that Colonel Tulloch would not be able to resist the temptation to have his day in court. He wrote to his assistant pointing out that their report was purely factual, and that if the officers who gave evidence now wanted to retract their signed statements that was the army's affair and he and Tulloch should not make any comment or try to defend their report. Tulloch should not attend the Generals' Board of Enquiry, because 'It would be a godsend to them to have an antagonist before the Board, and you could, not do them a greater favour than to place yourself in that position. Without an antagonist they will be firing in the air. The Press may perhaps try to provoke us to come forward for their own amusement and profit, but it will not do to be made sport for the Philistines. There is the Report, the evidence, and the other documents, that is all we have to say. Yours sincerely John McNeill.' But his worst fears were realised, and Tulloch set himself up before the Board as self-appointed prosecutor of the army, with the right to call and cross-examine witnesses.

The Board of Enquiry sat in the Royal Hospital at Chelsea. An old disabled soldier once accosted the kind hearted Nell Gwynne, mistress of King Charles II, and told her such a heartrending tale of hardship that she persuaded the king to found this retirement home for soldiers. It was a stately palace in thirty-six acres of parkland in what is now the heart of London. Sir Christopher Wren designed the building to combine economy of construction with monumental style, using high-quality brickwork with stone trimmings. In the Great Hall, a portrait of Charles II on horseback has looked down on the proceedings of many a court martial. It was here, in the heart of London's most military district, that the Board of Generals met in April 1856 to enquire into the very damaging statements made by McNeill and Tulloch about the conduct of certain senior army officers in the Crimea.

The enquiry quickly uncovered the government's pretence that they were only investigating the civilian Commissariat. Lord Lucan, who had been criticised, refused to answer a question from Colonel Tulloch on the grounds that it lay beyond the scope of the enquiry, having nothing to do with the Commissariat. Lord Lucan claimed: 'Having read the instructions most carefully and repeatedly, I have no hesitation in saying that I believe the object of those instructions was to confine your enquiry to the Commissariat supplies, and that you very much exceeded your duties when you went beyond it.' Colonel Tulloch responded by reading out the supplementary instructions to Lucan in front of the Board, showing that the government had instructed them to enquire into non-Commissariat stores. Until then the Army High Command seemed to be genuinely ignorant of the supplementary instructions published unobtrusively on the back of the main ones. Lucan now spectacularly lost his temper and began to rant incoherently about a conspiracy between Tulloch and the government.

Tulloch's appearance was a disaster, exactly as McNeill predicted. After several weeks of hostile interrogation the Colonel's health broke down and he had to withdraw. If the government had thought that the enquiry could trap the Board of Generals into approving the report's findings, they were wrong. As foreseen by McNeill and many others, the report of the Board found the army officers innocent of all the accusations, and put the blame on civilians in the Treasury at home instead. This conclusion was not surprising: Lord Hardinge, the home Commander-in-Chief and therefore the military superior of the Board's members, had already publicly denounced McNeill's report in the House of Lords, and it would have been hard for any of the Board to disagree with him.

The Board's report, which was a humiliating rebuff to McNeill and Tulloch, was presented to parliament just before the end of the session, in the summer of 1856. Shortly afterwards, Queen Victoria even persuaded the Cabinet to appoint her anti-reform cousin, the Duke of Cambridge, to be Commander-in-Chief of the army in place of Lord Hardinge. Hardinge had been in the midst of explaining the findings of the Board of Generals to Queen Victoria at Aldershot when he was cut down by a fatal stroke. When Florence Nightingale arrived back in England one month later, the whole affair seemed to be over and the reformers defeated.

It was not surprising that Nightingale decided to keep a low profile when she saw how pusillanimous the government had been and how a man as distinguished as her idol McNeill could be exposed to ridicule as a result. But within a few weeks, she had changed her mind again: she would campaign for reform, before returning to nursing. As well as ensuring that she would never work in a hospital again, this decision was to make Nightingale a key player in a continuing political crisis of which she was completely unaware. The squabble between the Army High Command and the Cabinet, and between Queen and parliament, for control of the Queen's Army was now nearing its climax.

Nightingale was first encouraged to enter the reform camp by her army sympathiser Colonel Lefroy when she asked him whether it would be dangerous for her to respond to the War Office's request that she answer some questions. His advice was that she should go much further and demand that the government authorise a public 'commission to enquire into the existing regulations for hospital administration'. She and others would then be able to give evidence to this commission on the Army Medical Department's brutal and incompetent treatment of sick and wounded soldiers, and the evidence would be published. She had never thought of a public enquiry before. Lefroy told her that an enquiry would be much more effective than giving her comments to the War Office in private as suggested by the civil servants. He also persuaded her that she was morally obliged to speak out, as the only person possessing the necessary information. Unknown to her, these suggestions were coming from the Cabinet itself. The Minister of War was frequently opposed by his own War Office bureaucrats, and the scheme that he instructed his reform-minded subordinate to implant in Nightingale's mind would enable him to outflank these civil servants, many of whom were too close to the Army High Command and were hostile to Nightingale. Just six weeks after her return, Florence Nightingale was invited to meet the Queen and the Prince Consort in Scotland, and she agreed to seek the Queen's support for a proposed 'Commission on Hospital Administration.'

She had not seen McNeill for more than twelve months, and she now wrote to him to invite herself to stay with him in Edinburgh so that he should tell her what subjects to raise with the Queen. McNeill used an unusually intimate salutation in his reply welcoming her to stay: *Dear Miss Florence*. This must have raised eyebrows when the letter was passed round the family as usual. Very few men outside the family addressed her by her first name. Sidney Herbert, for example, did not. It is unlikely that any of the family had met McNeill, and Bracebridge's indiscreet comment that McNeill had taken a great fancy to Nightingale was disturbing, especially because Florence had praised him to her family so effusively. On receiving McNeill's over familiar reply, Nightingale hurriedly cancelled her sleepover on a flimsy pretext, though she did meet him. Subsequent letters from McNeill begin *Dear Miss Nightingale*. If family reaction was behind this embarrassment it would not have been because of any suspicion of a love affair but rather a fear that McNeill was replacing her father in her affections. The incident is further evidence that their mutual affection was strong enough to be considered inappropriate. She did stay with McNeill on later occasions.

Her letters recounting her meeting with the Queen show that she found the Prince sympathetic to her criticisms, although she was 'somewhat alarmed at his predilection for the Horse Guards' – meaning that she found that the Prince was on the side of the Army High Command. She had no way of knowing in advance that Victoria and Albert at this time would have been horrified at the thought of another public commission investigating army blunders. She knew nothing of the disagreement between Monarch and Cabinet, and did not realise that the Royal couple's deep interest in her story was due to their belief that if the health of the army had been neglected it was a matter for the Queen's Ministers to put right in private. Nightingale thought it was Lord Panmure and his fellow aristocrats in the army who had 'herded together' to use the Board of Generals to bury McNeill's report two months previously. She had little confidence in the idea of a public enquiry, thinking that it would fail because army witnesses would be afraid to speak out after the McNeill debacle. She therefore planned to suggest to the Queen that she make a confidential report to

Her Majesty, bypassing Lord Panmure. But when she talked this over with the Queen, Nightingale's interest in making a confidential report to Her Majesty evaporated. She also concluded that the Queen would not be of much use in persuading the Minister of War to initiate a public enquiry. Perhaps Victoria was a little too open with Nightingale about her anger that the Cabinet had allowed McNeill's report to be published.

Lord Palmerston, the Prime Minister, then sent Nightingale a message asking her to make a confidential report to the Cabinet on the war and begging her to stay at Balmoral until Lord Panmure arrived so that she could try to convince the War Minister of the necessity for army reform. Coming from the politician and friend whom her father most admired, Palmerston's appeal must have finally convinced her that it was her duty to fight for reform, and reinforced her belief that the War Minister was an opponent to be won over. In early October 1856, Nightingale met Lord Panmure with the Queen at Balmoral and then alone nearby. Panmure agreed 'in principle' to appoint a royal commission along the lines that Nightingale wanted. Panmure arranged to meet her privately in London the following month to discuss details of the proposed Royal Commission. He also confirmed that the Cabinet wanted a confidential report from her.

Nightingale moved into the Burlington Hotel, in Mayfair, early in November 1856 to begin work on the confidential report to the Cabinet which she hoped would also form the evidence to be submitted to the Royal Commission. Two weeks later, the Minster of War called on her there. They discussed her proposed list of experts to sit on the commission, and she was surprised and pleased that she persuaded Lord Panmure to accept so many reformers. But without a major political upheaval there was not the remotest chance that the government could appoint a Royal Commission in the face of the Queen's and the Duke of Cambridge's certain opposition, least of all with the wide-ranging scope and the slate of reform-minded commissioners that Lord Panmure had now promised Nightingale. The military lobby in parliament, together with Palmerston's other rivals, was strong enough to command a majority and bring down the government. Nightingale believed that the lack of progress was caused by divisions within the Cabinet, and as the weeks went by she began to write her confidential report, determined to publish it if necessary.

She wrote to McNeill asking him to give her material to include in her confidential report, and suggestions for improving hospital management structure, cost control, division of labour, and statistical reporting. McNeill helped her to introduce into her report many of his own findings on the army's mistreatment of its men. Nightingale also contacted Colonel Tulloch, who was now writing a book exposing the untruths in the report of the Board of Generals. One remarkable feature of Tulloch's book was soon to prove extremely important to Nightingale. This was the table of sickness and mortality that the Colonel had compiled in the Crimea on his own initiative, which the government had suppressed because of its potential impact on morale while the war was still continuing. Now that the war was over, Tulloch published it in his book for the first time in January 1857. He may have showed it to Nightingale a month or so before; she wrote to McNeill in December 1856 criticising the book for being too vehement.

Tulloch was a desk colonel who had made a name for himself in India through his hobby of compiling statistics and extracting useful information from them. He showed great ingenuity in collecting sickness and mortality data for the troops on foreign stations. He noticed from his statistics that there was a remarkable tendency for military pensioners to live to extreme old age, and on investigation he was able to show that relatives of deceased soldiers were concealing their deaths so as to continue to draw the pension. Tulloch also exposed a number of frauds that the East India Company were practising on the common soldiers by depriving them of their pay and forcing them to buy goods at extortionate prices.

Nightingale agreed with McNeill that Tulloch was too vehement and intolerant of other peoples' ideas. He and McNeill were probably not on speaking terms any more, because at the disastrous Board of Enquiry Tulloch had produced a private letter that McNeill had written him, and it was published in the newspapers. McNeill wrote him a reprimand for this breach of trust that was so savage that it would be hard for the two ever to be reconciled. Despite Tulloch's indiscretion, Nightingale recognised and admired his genuine interest in the troops' welfare. No sooner had he arrived in the Crimea than he was up to his elbows in flour, baking bread for the soldiers who had been living up to then on salt meat and hard biscuit. She described him with a word that was probably one of the highest compliments in her vocabulary: 'Tulloch was, in one sense, a kind of Deliverer, and McNeill is a far better man.' It was a common literary device of Nightingale's to describe someone using both an extravagant compliment and a slight put-down incongruously in the same sentence, to catch the reader's attention and demonstrate her objectivity. To rank McNeill above 'Deliverer' was a rare compliment.

One of the reasons for earlier friction between McNeill and Tulloch had been the latter's objection to McNeill's adulation of Nightingale. He objected to McNeill's praise of Scutari hospital and of Nightingale in the draft of their report. 'I much doubt the expediency of our going into the details of that Hospital at all, but if we do, I submit it should not be in positive terms . . . I now come to the paragraph about Miss Nightingale. No one is disposed to admire more than I do her devotion and courage, but I doubt whether the place to allude to it is in a parliamentary report ... Does this not rather look like being partisans? I felt so strongly the necessity of not expressing my opinions or feelings in any way regarding Miss Nightingale and her assistants, that I refused to be one of the Committee [of the Nightingale Fund, set up by Sidney Herbert the previous month] or take any hand in the arrangements for the Subscription, till I was clear of this report, that I might not be suspected of any bias either way.' McNeill removed the paragraphs that Tulloch objected to.

Tulloch agreed with McNeill that, as the opening page of their report said, 'the sick arriving [at Scutari] from the Crimea were nearly all suffering from diseases chiefly attributable to diet.' But his reluctance to praise the Scutari hospital stemmed from his belief that some of the patients might have contracted other more fatal diseases in the hospital itself. This he made clear on the last page of his own book, but it was also probably his idea to include the following paragraph in his and McNeill's report twelve months earlier: 'The mortality in the whole army was further increased by the diseases which broke out at Scutari . . . Had the sanitary condition of these establishments been from the first what it afterwards became, there can be little doubt that the mortality would have been perceptibly reduced.' If Tulloch expressed this opinion when he returned to England, it might have been the reason that Nightingale felt it necessary to write to the Minister of War two months later denying that the 'Scutari air' had contributed to the death of her patients, and claiming that the reason for the lower mortality later was that the men were now being sent in time to be saved.

If there was anyone who knew about what we now call 'hospital acquired infection' at that time, it was Tulloch's friend and statistical mentor Dr William Farr, and that may be why Tulloch advised Nightingale to meet him in case he could contribute some statistics for her report. Nothing could be less descriptive of the spirit of the extraordinary Dr Farr than his dour Victorian title: Superintendent of the Statistical Department of the Registrar-General's Office. The broad scope of Farr's genius owed much to his varied background and early career. His parents were illiterate labourers known to a horse-drawn cab driver from Bath named Price who had saved a modest cash sum from his labours. Price recognised an unusual talent in their son and apprenticed him to an apothecary. When Farr was 21, Price died and left him £500. Farr used the hoarded cab fares to travel to Paris and study a most unusual subject in the Paris Medical School: hygiene. He set up in practice in London but found that his humble background was a handicap that the science of hygiene was considered a threat by the medical establishment. No medical school would allow him to teach the subject in England, and he became a medical journalist instead, advocating reform of the medical profession. He published articles promoting the use of medical statistics to advance public health, and when the General Register Office was set up he was taken onto the staff.

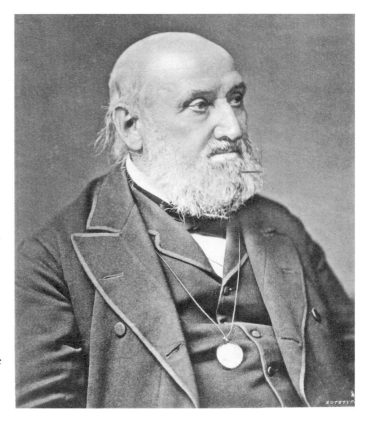

William Farr, the chief statistician at the General Registry Office.

For the first time births, marriages, and deaths were systematically recorded, and from the start Farr was responsible for writing the explanations to accompany the summarised statistics produced in the Office. He built a reputation both for his skill with numbers and his ability to extract inspirational conclusions from them, for the quality of his 'Biometers' or Life Tables showing the deaths per thousand at each age group, and for the insight he provided into how the 'life force' of the population might be prolonged through public health measures. His vision was of a future world where nearly everyone lived to a maximum life span, not through advances in curative medicine but through prevention of epidemic diseases which, he believed, weakened the survivors at the same time as directly causing many premature deaths. Epidemic disease was largely responsible for the fact that life expectancy was less than forty years in Britain. 'If the secret roots of death were once pointed out by authentic observation,' Farr wrote, in his habitual lyrical style, 'the human frame might be prolonged to its full ripeness, until it fell as gently as a plant upon the earth.'

On 24 November 1856, Nightingale had a first momentous meeting with Farr at the General Registry Office at Somerset House, and wrote a note describing her visit:

Through the kindness of the Registrar-General, went over with him all his books . . .

When one business-like head sets out to accomplish one object, if that object is to make beer we see the results in, say, the Burton Breweries. When one mathematical head sets out to accomplish one object, that of classifying and registering the great statistics and discovering the causes of the various events in a population we see the results in a magnificent organisation, magnificent because of its simplicity, economy, and efficiency in the Registrar-General's office.

A weekly published return, such as the Registrar General's office gives, of disease, might have saved our Army . . . The Government could hardly, in face of such information, have gone on supplying us with salt meat and biscuit . . . In January 1855, losing at the rate of 576 per 1000, corresponding week of January 1856 rate of 17 per 1000. The more I think of these things, the more I feel both the absolute necessity of ripping up our army system and the impossibility (almost) of your gaining evidence to do so.

This note is rich in social commentary. Her comparison between the General Registry Office's efficient mass production of statistics and the Burton Breweries' prodigiously efficient mass-production of beer shows that the methods of the industrial revolution had inspired changes in civil government, and marks the awakening of her desire to transfer these methods to military affairs. She now believes that timely Crimean statistics would have proved that men were dying in her hospital because of poor food rations in the Crimea. The appearance of the mortality statistics of the Scutari hospitals in the middle of the note suggests that Farr actually calculated them for her during the course of this visit to Somerset House – the beginning of her new education.

Exactly how many men had died in the war Nightingale did not know, and even when Colonel Tulloch shared his statistics with her they covered only seven months of the two-year conflict. In her letters written after returning to England she often mentioned various total numbers of dead, but without making clear whether the numbers were supposed to refer to deaths in her Turkish hospitals or in the whole of the war zone. Nightingale was obviously quoting vague estimates from different sources without a clear definition of what was included. The army did not publish its official statistics until twelve months later. By that time Nightingale had long abandoned the practice of quoting vague numbers; she had appointed herself guardian of the Crimean mortality figures and treated them as sacred relics never to be exhibited without their full statistical regalia and provenance. The foundations of her statistical treatment were laid in her work with Farr in the winter of 1856/57.

But Farr was much more than a statistician, and statistical wisdom was not all that Nightingale took away from that first momentous meeting. Farr was the apostle of hygiene, the prophet of the sanitarian movement which urged the expenditure of public funds on sewers, clean water, and ventilation of dwellings, the friend of Dr John Sutherland who had led the Sanitary Commission to Scutari and had put the sanitation to rights in Nightingale's hospital with the minimum of fuss. Nightingale wrote a letter on the same day to Lady Canning, one of her pre-war hospital committee members, in which she shows more respect for Sutherland's commission than before. Although (as seen in her note above) she still thinks that poor diet before admission to hospital was the main killer, Farr must have told her that Sutherland's efforts had at least reduced the mortality from cholera: 'Deaths from Epidemics were reduced from 70 per cent of those from all causes to 45 per cent . . . This of course, is attributable to the excellent sanitary arrangements in the Army, introduced by the Sanitary Commission . . . The frightful mortality in the Barrack Hospital at Scutari diminished in like manner. During 54-55, that Hospital was literally living over a cess-pool – & the Military Medical Officers ascribed the unmanageable outbreaks of Cholera which took place up to November 1855 to a Cemetery 3/4 mile off -!!'

In this letter to Lady Canning, she makes clear what she means by the word 'sanitation'. She lists sixteen recommendations that she proposes to make in her report, eleven of which relate to the army outside the hospitals and mostly deal with supplies, and mentions sanitation twice. She defines it thus: 'a sanitary officer . . . to advise on matters relating to encampment, diet, clothing, hutting, sick transport.' This definition is consistent with the 1842 *Inquiry into the Sanitary Conditions of the Labouring Population*, when it meant (as its classical root indicates) simply *health care*. Since then specialists like Farr and Sutherland had given the word a much more modern meaning, using it to refer to that part of health care that is concerned with cleanliness. Sutherland's Sanitary Commission, for example, had not concerned itself with matters of diet and clothing. Nightingale's use of the word would soon change, under the influence of Farr and Sutherland.

By early 1857, Nightingale was smouldering with fury at the government's failure to set up the promised Royal Commission of Enquiry, and she told McNeill that she planned to leak her confidential report to the public so as to reopen the debate into his findings which had been buried by the Generals. But Palmerston had by now given McNeill a personal guarantee that he would eventually be vindicated. McNeill had also become convinced of the government's sincerity when he learned that they did everything possible to dissuade the excitable Colonel Tulloch from appearing at the Generals' Enquiry. If the government had wanted to discredit McNeill, as the public assumed they did, they would have encouraged him to take this foolish step. So Sir John persuaded Nightingale to be patient because he believed that, under a calm surface, Palmerston had a plan. He was right; the plan involved using the parliamentary recess in the autumn of 1856 to lobby public opinion against the Board of Generals' report. Not through the newspapers, but through personal contacts with influential citizens throughout the country. The Board of Generals' report must have been a best seller, because when parliament reconvened at the beginning of 1857, every prominent citizen in the country seemed to have formed an opinion on it. It was not for nothing that Palmerston had wholeheartedly approved the Queen's proposal to revive the 1808 precedent of a Generals' Enquiry. She had not realised that the report of the 1808 enquiry had been published, but Palmerston had been well aware of this detail. Amazingly, he had already been in the government half a century before as a Navy Minister. Queen Victoria would have had to get up very early in the morning to outsmart Lord Palmerston.

It might have been better for the Queen if she and the Army High Command had simply ignored McNeill's critical report. Peace was then breaking out in the Crimea and the army would emerge with some credit: the public had no way of knowing whether the defects exposed had now been corrected. But now the people could see for themselves how the Generals had whitewashed their colleagues, how Lord Lucan had ranted and raved at poor Tulloch, and how the chief culprits had been promoted and handsomely rewarded by the Army High Command and by the Queen. The electorate now made its views known through a series of ceremonial public addresses to Sir John McNeill and Colonel Tulloch, signed by mayors, aldermen, councillors, magistrates, and other worthies of the manufacturing towns. These addresses thanked McNeill and Tulloch in the most fulsome terms, and castigated parliament for failing to do the same.

Liverpool was the first, noting in January 1857 that although 'honours have been bestowed upon some of those to whom the sad calamities which occurred were mainly owing, the honest exertion you made to retrieve, in some degree, those disasters, have so far been treated with cold neglect'. Ignored by a supine parliament, the services of the two Crimean commissioners were nevertheless 'cherished in the affections of a grateful nation'. After Liverpool came Preston, and then a tide of high-flown compliments swept the two commissioners onto the nation's pedestal as the gowns, wigs, and chains of office rose to be counted in the richest towns in the land. Liverpool, Preston, Bath, Edinburgh, Manchester, Birmingham, all declared themselves for McNeill and Tulloch and against the Army High Command. It was impossible, said one municipal address, to decide which was the stronger emotion felt in contemplating both McNeill's report and that of the Board of Generals: was it pride at the first, or shame at the second? And it is equally impossible, seeing these addresses following so closely on one another, to believe that there was not some co-ordination among them.

The House of Commons did its best to ignore the opprobrium heaped on it by the country's civic leaders. According to Nightingale, who by this time had given up hope of reform, the pro-army lobby in parliament was strong enough to prevent the government from acting. She thought that Palmerston had missed his chance the previous summer, when he still could have called a general election on the issue: 'Eight months ago,' she wrote on 1 March, 'had Lord Palmerston chosen to play a great game and say "I will have Army Reform, and if the House of Commons is against me, let me see if the country is for me", he might have won. Now it is too late. The opportunity is lost and we shall not see another in our lifetime. The Army is strong enough now in the House of Commons to turn out any Ministry as it always has been in the House of Lords . . . Had Lord Palmerston been a younger man, this never could have happened.'

But she was wrong. At the age of seventy-three, Palmerston was not quite over the hill. In accordance with the Queen's wishes, he continued to resist the demands of the House that he publicly honour the two neglected commissioners, and was even dismissive of the value of McNeill's report whereas previously he had praised it. This public about-face did not perturb McNeill, who tried to calm his more ardent supporters by hinting to one of them that a theatrical performance was in progress: 'There seems to be a general impression among the Members of Parliament that Lord Palmerston spoke under some kind of restraint and difficulty – that there was some unseen influence which he could not overcome.' This unseen influence was obviously emanating from Buckingham Palace.

The government then made an insulting offer of £1,000 each to McNeill and Tulloch, evidently a Royal idea that the government eagerly adopted to teach Buckingham Palace a lesson. The thought of being governed by people who believed that this was the most proper way to reward this type of public service was enough to make the electorate's collective cheeks burn with shame. The House of Commons, far from agreeing that the proposed reward made a debate unnecessary, now united in demanding one. In the debate, Palmerston goaded the House to fury by making further disparaging comments about McNeill and Tulloch. It was left to Sidney Herbert to propose the motion that Her Majesty should be asked to confer a more appropriate reward. No more members could speak because shouts for a vote on the motion were so loud, and it was obvious that the government would be massively defeated if it did not act.

Palmerston, relieved that the House had finally done its duty and listened to the voice of the people, yielded with a show of displeasure. Within days he gave Tulloch a knighthood. Sir John McNeill, who had received a knighthood for service in Persia, declined the offer to convert it into a baronetcy (inheritable by the male line) because he now only had a daughter and instead was made a member of the Privy Council, the highest policymaking body in the land. This gave him the title of The Right Honourable. Sir Alexander Tulloch was gratified that the War Minister sent for him to give him a personal apology, telling him that there had been great difficulties that he could not explain.

A few days later, Palmerston tricked his opponents into defeating him in a vote in the House on a quite different matter. He told the Queen that he was obliged to call a general election as a result and the Queen granted the request, hoping to be rid of him. But the electorate returned him and his party to power in a landslide which swept the opposition party and the military lobby into oblivion. There began a parliamentary session of such tranquillity that the gossipy political diarist Greville was almost in despair: 'June 3rd [1857]. There is really nothing to write about, but it is evident that the session is going to pass away in a most quiet and uneventful manner. Never had Minister such a peaceful and undisturbed reign as Palmerston's. There is something almost alarming in his prodigious felicity and success. Everything prospers with him. In the House of Commons there is scarcely a semblance of opposition to anything he proposes; a speech or two here and there from some stray Radical, against some part of the Princess Royal's dowry, but hardly any attempt at division; and when there have been any, the minorities have been so ridiculously small as to show the hopelessness of opposition.'

Shortly after the election, Palmerston's War Minister turned up at the Burlington Hotel bringing Nightingale the thing she most desired, which he would have had great difficulty in giving her before the military lobby in parliament had been cut down to size: the agreed instructions for the Royal Commission into the Sanitary Condition of the Army. The instructions were virtually unchanged from her proposed draft.

It is not clear whether Nightingale was properly able to savour this victory because at almost exactly the same time her work with Farr on Tulloch's wartime mortality statistics had led to a startling conclusion. An analysis of the differences between the mortality in different areas, and specifically between the regimental hospitals in the Crimea and the general hospitals at Scutari in the first winter, had convinced Farr that the disease that had killed 16,000 men out of an army intended to number 25,000 had *not* been caused by inadequate diet before admission to hospital. Neither was it due to overwork or exposure as some believed. Not only cholera, but virtually all fatal disease had been caused by bad sanitation. The worst affected places had been those where overcrowding had aggravated the effect of poor hygiene. And by far the worst of these, where 5,000 men had been killed by bad sanitation in the winter of 1854/55, was Florence Nightingale's hospital complex near Constantinople. In the five months before the Sanitary Commission arrived, between November 1854 and March 1855, Farr's statistics showed that Nightingale had not been running a hospital. She had been running a death camp.

CHAPTER FIVE

Conversion

It took months for Farr to convince her, and for Nightingale to admit that she had been wrong. But was it true? The statistics do seem to show that sick soldiers were better off in their muddy hospital marquees at the front, bare of medicines, than in her grand hospital buildings with their well-organised nurses and their civilian doctors recruited from the best schools in Europe. But it is hard to see how Farr's statistics could be reliable, some of them apparently gathered from memory two years after the fact. And wasn't the ultimate cause of death still the poor diet, because without that the soldiers either wouldn't have been in hospital at all or wouldn't have been so susceptible to the diseases they caught after admission?

The answer to these questions lies in the political context. Simple numbers and pure facts do not turn someone into a fervent disciple or a visionary – there needs to be a political dimension to the facts. When someone has bought into the political message, the limitations in the evidence and the existence of other perspectives become simply distractions, obstacles to be overcome.

Sir John McNeill had given Nightingale a political angle: he showed her that the aristocratic officers looked on the common soldier as an inferior species. This was not so eccentric of them when one takes into account the ideas prevailing at the time – even Charles Darwin believed in the inheritance of acquired characteristics and favoured the annihilation of inferior races. That wasn't what Nightingale believed with her well-developed social conscience and her religious faith in the perfectibility of the common man; McNeill's outrage resonated with her already well-developed social philosophy. She came to see herself as McNeill's lieutenant in a campaign to reform the British Army, and this did not conflict with her original mission of proving that women could be organised into an effective workforce in hospitals.

This is why Nightingale paid little attention to any claim that there might be a problem with the Scutari hospitals. The improved survival rate, she claimed during the war, was only due to the fact that 'The men sent down to Scutari in the winter died because they were not sent down till half dead – the men sent down now live and recover because they are sent in time.' But one letter that she wrote during the war to Lady Cranworth, a member of her Harley Street Committee, seems to admit that hospital conditions might have played a role: 'They [the French] tell the same story that we did last year – that want of food and clothing sends down the patients in a typhoid state which is propagated by the overcrowded state of the hospitals.' This is a detached view of things, not attributing any fault to the hospital itself but rather regarding hospital acquired infection as something that 'goes with the territory', being caused by the patients themselves – not an unusual position even today. This was at a time when McNeill's report was being debated in London, and for Nightingale the army's supply defects were the main issue. The idea that there might be fatalities due to hospital conditions had no political implications at all for her at that time.

This changed when she discovered after the war, when working with Farr and Sutherland, why the buildings at Scutari had not been inspected by sanitation experts before being used as a hospital. She learned that the Sanitary Commission had arrived at Scutari six months late because it had been delayed by politics. The commission's secret instigator was a figure who at that time was politically unpopular throughout England for his dictatorial approach to public health: the disgraced would-be sanitary czar Edwin Chadwick.

Chadwick's movement to clean up London and other cities in England, which had begun with the passing of the Public Health Act in 1848, had run out of steam in 1854 a few months before Nightingale went to the Crimea. That summer, parliament abolished the General Board of Health, which had been created in 1848 under a previous Liberal government. The Board of Health had been led by Chadwick, who was Secretary of the Poor Law Commission, and Lord Shaftesbury, President of the Health of Towns Association.

Chadwick despised medical science. He believed that sanitary administration was a matter for engineers and lawyers. 'Sanitary Science' according to Chadwick, was 'a subsidiary department of engineering, a science with which medical practitioners could have little or nothing to do.' Not surprisingly, the medical profession joined with many vested interests to oppose the spending of public money on Chadwick's expensive sewerage and water supply projects. The main losers from his schemes were property owners, who would have to pay for the improvements through local taxes. At the time, only property owners could vote in parliamentary elections so it was not hard for the anti-Chadwick faction to impose their will on the government, claiming that Chadwick's aim was to take money from the pockets of the rich and give it to builders, plumbers, and overpaid government inspectors.

Edwin Chadwick was a public relations disaster. He tried to give the impression that his great humanitarian schemes could only work if he alone was in absolute charge, and he always talked in pounds, shillings, and pence rather than in human terms. With an air of goggle-eyed contempt for their stupidity, he would bore his audiences rigid with theoretical calculations of how his proposed municipal piped water schemes would, by bringing soft water to the cities, save thousands of pounds worth of soap. Only the soap manufacturers would get excited by such calculations, and then in the wrong direction.

Chadwick's strongest supporter in parliament had been Lord Palmerston, who as Home Secretary was closely concerned with the Board of Health, but in 1854 his speech in defence of Chadwick was to no avail. When parliament voted the Board out of existence and sacked Chadwick and his employees, *The Times* voiced its readers' relief. 'Mr Chadwick has been deposed, and we prefer to take our chance of cholera and the rest, than to be bullied into health.'

Early in the war, Chadwick told Palmerston that sanitation was being neglected by the Army High Command, and Palmerston tried to persuade the Duke of Newcastle, who shared responsibility for military affairs with Sidney Herbert, to send out a civilian commission to look into the

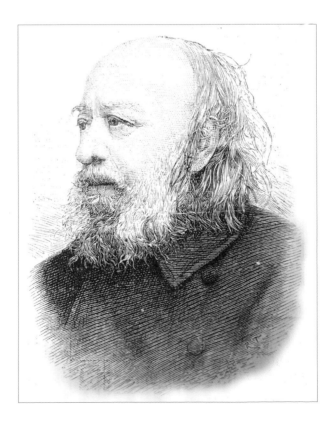

Edwin Chadwick.

problem. His suggestion was rejected. But when Palmerston became Prime Minister three months after Nightingale went to the East, Chadwick's influence made itself felt immediately. Palmerston wrote to his War Minister on his first day in office telling him to send Chadwick's most trusted experts to sort out a problem in Nightingale's hospital. His letter shows that Palmerston was extremely well-informed about the sanitation there, a problem that was to receive no mention at all in the House of Commons' Sebastopol Enquiry which was getting under way. Palmerston wrote to his new Minister of War:

> It is clear that, quite independently of the medical treatment of the sick and wounded, there is an urgent necessity for improved sanitary arrangements in our hospitals at Constantinople, Scutari, and elsewhere. Proper ventilation has been neglected, and various other sanitary arrangements have been either not thought of, or not carried into effect.
>
> There are two very able and active men who have been connected with the Board of Health and whom I have much employed about sanitary matters – Dr Sutherland and Dr Grainger. I wish very much that you would send them out at once to Constantinople, and one afterwards to Scutari and Balaclava and the Camp, not to interfere at all with the medical treatment of the sick and wounded, but with full powers to carry into immediate effect such sanitary improvements and arrangements in regard to the hospital buildings and to the Camp as their experience may suggest. I am convinced that this will save a great many lives.

This letter shows that there must have already been debate about sanitation problems at Scutari under the previous government, but no action had been taken. Florence Nightingale never found out about this letter otherwise she would not later have given so much credit to Lord Shaftesbury, the great Victorian philanthropist, for sending out the Sanitary Commission. Shaftesbury, Lord Palmerston's son-in-law, did propose a commission but not until three days after Palmerston sent the above instructions. Shaftesbury submitted to Palmerston a different proposed list of sanitary experts to form the commission including John Simon, the anti-Chadwick Health Officer of the City of London. By the time the commission was ready to sail, however, John Simon had been replaced by one of Chadwick's engineers.

It seems likely that Chadwick himself proposed the final list of names of his commissioners to Lord Palmerston and persuaded the Prime Minister to pass over John Simon, but Chadwick could not stop his rival's rapid rise to power. John Simon was a well-connected surgeon and pathologist of conservative political views; by the end of the war he was the Chief Medical Officer to the new Board of Health. His high-tech medical and scientific theories of public health were in complete opposition to Chadwick's theory that sanitary science was 'a subsidiary department of engineering'. John Simon had risen to prominence in the only corner of England where Chadwick's power had never held sway: the City of London.

In 1848, the City of London Corporation had refused to allow its opulent but filthy Square Mile to be incorporated into Chadwick's sanitary empire. 'That nasty turtle-eating Corporation,' as a contemporary MP described it, had obtained its own Act of Parliament to regulate its sanitation independently. To buttress its independence, the City of London Corporation had appointed its own salaried Medical Officer, and this was John Simon's first public appointment. Simon had impeccable political and technical credentials. His father was a member of one of the City Livery Companies and a prominent member of the Committee of the London Stock Exchange. Simon himself was a respected surgeon, and had become a Fellow of the Royal Society at a young age through his research in pathology. When a national Chief Medical Officer was appointed to replace Chadwick, Simon was the obvious choice.

The members of the Crimean Sanitary Commission, Robert Rawlinson, John Sutherland, and Hector Gavin, had all worked for Chadwick at the General Board of Health. Rawlinson was an engineer, and Sutherland

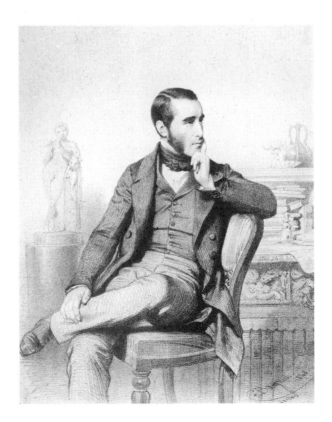

John Simon, Chief Medical Officer of Health.

and Gavin were doctors who had converted to Chadwick's non-medical approach. In sending them, the Prime Minister was undermining the new high-tech medical approach of John Simon and reviving the Chadwick movement. William Farr was also a part of that movement; he owed his job at the Registry Office in part to Chadwick, whose most famous contribution to setting up the registry system was the idea of including the cause of death in the returns.

Hector Gavin, the second doctor on the Sanitary Commission, had already written extensively on health matters and would certainly have become one of the great figures of Victorian sanitary reform. He was accidentally shot dead by his brother William, a veterinary surgeon in the 17th Lancers, after only six weeks in the East. Robert Rawlinson, who was to become one of Britain's most eminent engineers, had to go home after he visited the front and was struck a glancing blow by one of the endless shower of Russian cannon balls that bounced through the British lines. This left Dr Sutherland, a rather colourless individual with a short attention span, to sort out the mess with the Inspectors of Nuisances from Liverpool. They were exactly what was needed. Sutherland stayed in Scutari and the Crimea for the duration of the war and made himself indispensable to Nightingale as her personal physician and advisor. He was inclined to avoid confrontation, to Nightingale's later disappointment, but his conciliatory approach enabled him to get cooperation from the army doctors in his sanitary improvements.

Nightingale's post-war mentor William Farr was a different matter, a controversial and confrontational medical reformer who had an axe to grind because his studies of environmental hygiene were given a hostile reception by the medical profession. Farr approached Nightingale's Crimean mortality problem with a prejudice: he believed that armies were a laboratory in which one could prove the relative uselessness of doctors and hospitals. He had been very impressed at the Paris Medical School years before by studies of the sickness and mortality of armies that showed that different hygiene practices, not medical treatments, accounted for all known differences in army mortality. This had led him to try to demonstrate that hospitals themselves could spread disease, and that bigger hospitals were worse in this respect. His investigation had failed because of poor hospital statistics which made it impossible to tell whether the bigger hospitals had a higher death rate because they were accepting a worse class of patients than the others. As it happened, Farr had helped Tulloch in his confrontation with the Generals, trying to show by statistical analysis that Lord Lucan had allowed his cavalry horses to starve to death. When Nightingale asked Dr Farr to investigate the mortality statistics of the war to see whether he could prove that the army had similarly mistreated its men, Farr saw it as an opportunity to test his own theories instead.

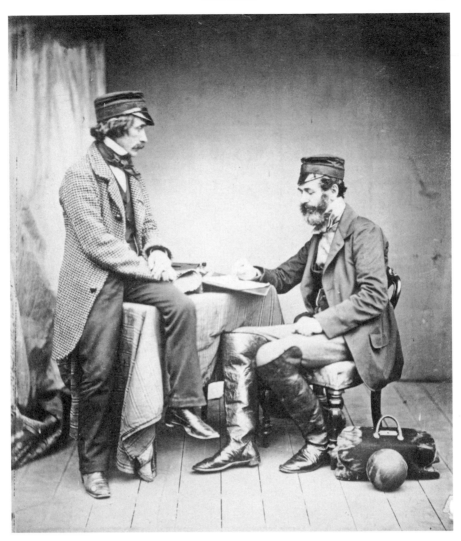

Dr John Sutherland and Robert Rawlinson, Sanitary Commissioners. Rawlinson is displaying the Russian cannonball which wounded him.

Farr's theory of sanitation was based on the unproven and controversial belief that some diseases could spread through either the atmosphere or the water supply by some chemical means. This explained why the diseases spread more easily in crowded environments and large buildings. He was using what were at that time relatively advanced notions of chemistry to explain why defensive sanitary measures worked – they removed the offending substances from a contaminated environment. This was not related to the so-called 'miasmatic' theory that diseases had their *origin* in, and spontaneously evolved out of, decaying matter. Farr's theory was about transmission, not origin. It contrasted with the 'contagionist' theory, which was then in vogue with most medical men, which held that most disease was transmitted only through direct physical contact – as implied by the classical derivation of the word – so that environmental improvements could not stop disease spreading. Farr's idea was closer to the germ theory, which would not start to achieve respectability until a decade later. Because 'contagion' now also refers to environmental transmission by germs, many people are misled into thinking that John Simon and his colleagues were already into germ theory, but that was still in the future.

Farr could now explain to Nightingale how political interests had derailed Chadwick's environmental approach to preventive medicine. He saw that the conversion of Nightingale to his beliefs would be an important breakthrough. Her family was on terms of friendship with the political aristocracy – they visited the Prime Minister at his home that Christmas – and Farr might now have a champion who could speak for him in circles from which his own humble background and lowly bureaucratic status excluded him. Although Nightingale referred to him as the 'Registrar General', that sinecure position was actually occupied by a well-born nonentity; Farr's colleagues thought this unjust and were kind enough to bestow the title on him unofficially.

For at least two months, Nightingale tried to persuade Farr that the army had starved the soldiers to death. Farr, probably aided by his friend Colonel Tulloch who had always harboured suspicions about the Scutari hospitals, sought more statistics from the regimental surgeons. Meanwhile, Nightingale's drafts of her confidential report still blamed the army for sending to hospital what we might call with modern irony 'the wrong type of patient'. On the 24th February, three months after starting to work with Farr, she wrote to a family friend bewailing the persecution of McNeill and Tulloch by the aristocratic Army High Command: 'the disgraceful triumph of all the Staff who neglected & lost the Army & their being put in high places – the deliberate persecution of the men who told the truth & saved the Army . . . I prophesy that the real effect & only lasting one of all this will be the sapping of the power of the aristocracy in the minds of the people of England, though historians will not perhaps trace the cause . . .'

Evidently, from her use of the word 'persecution' she still held that McNeill's Supplies Commission, and his fresh meat and fresh bread, had saved the second army sent to the East. But conflicting messages had begun to emerge from the statistics that Farr was gathering from barracks at home which showed that soldiers, although selected from the general population for their greater fitness, were dying younger because their barracks were less hygienic than the surrounding districts. *They* were not suffering any supply shortages, nor were they living on salt meat and biscuit. So there was something in Farr's theory. And in hindsight, there were things that happened at Scutari that only Farr could explain.

The fatal beds, for one. The nurses kept telling her that the patients put in certain beds always died quicker. And those healthy discharged soldiers, on their way back to England, who were lodged in the wards of the Scutari hospital while they waited for their ships home. And that perfectly clean English railway workman, in a Sunday-best top hat, who came in feeling a little unwell. He had come out to the East on a contract to make a little money because his savings bank had gone bust and he had orphaned grandchildren to support. He thought that if he earned a little from helping to build the army's railway he would not have to worry that his wife and companion of forty years might end up in the workhouse. But healthy discharged soldiers and tidy workman alike were tumbled in to a common grave with the human wrecks from the trenches, and at home the workhouse opened its cheerless arms to their loved ones.

Yes, there *had* been a problem. There *was* something in Farr's theory. Late in March she was admitting as much to her father, and showing that Farr's ideas had taken on a spiritual significance. Her father wrote to her sorrowfully announcing that he had not been selected as a parliamentary candidate in Palmerston's opportunistic general election: 'You, my only genius!' he wrote, 'You might have been my prompter and my supporter in political life. But no . . . Shall we have a House of Commons in the next life?' His daughter's magisterial reply is more like that of a parent to a child: 'Dearest Pa, I am sorry that you will not enter the House of Commons in this world. But I am very sure that there is a House of Commons in the next. I hope one upon sounder principles . . . Do you believe that He stops the fever, in answer not to "From plague, pestilence and famine, Good Lord, deliver us" but to His word and thought being carried out in a drain, a pipe-tile, a washhouse?'

She was aligning herself with Farr, under his patient tutoring. A rare insight into their interaction comes from a charming vignette written by her sister Parthe:

All of a sudden she said 'I have been looking into the Camp Regulations. What is the number of living souls in a square mile of London?' '23,000 generally, 30 or 40,000 perhaps in the very thickest parts,' said Farr. She replied: 'The disposition of tents by the Quarter Master General's order is thus: [diagram] back to back and touching! . . . one million one hundred thousand men to the square mile, I write it in figures so that you may not mistake. The French and the Sardinians are not such fools, we only (for strategical reasons of course they will say but really from sheer ignorance) treat our men thus; think of it being left to Miss F N, young lady, in 1857, to discover this.

Parthe added proudly: 'Farr calls it her greatest feat & when one sees such things one does not wonder at her risking life & health to right such wrongs.'

The tipping point came when Farr received some new statistics, presumably from regimental surgeons, which allowed them to compare the death rate at Scutari to that in the regimental hospitals. In those first terrible six months after her arrival, 12,000 patients came to her. They were mostly sick, not wounded, transferred from primitive regimental hospitals at the front where one in eight would have died. Among those sent to Nightingale's hospital, where medical supplies and skill were relatively plentiful but the men were packed like sardines in an unventilated building on top of defective sewers, instead of one in eight dying it became three in eight. A significant proportion died on the ships, but her hospital was easily twice as lethal even without the voyage. And the transfers into her hospital had continued, month after month, while nobody noticed.

At first, she tried not to let go of the explanation that she publicly committed herself to before meeting Farr. He was right, the hospitals were lethal but so was the cruel starvation. If the army had treated the men properly they wouldn't have ended up in those deadly hospitals. She wrote at the end of March to Sir John McNeill, arranging a visit to him to discuss her new findings, mentioning 'a system which, in the Crimea, put to death 16,000 men, the finest experiment modern history has seen upon a large scale viz. as to what given number may be put to death at will by the sole agency of bad food and bad air.'

But the 'bad food *and* bad air' formula didn't really work for her. You can't run a lethal hospital, she realised, and then cast a portion of the blame for it on the people who send you the patients. Quite distinct areas of culpability must exist for faults outside and inside the hospital respectively. A new thought crystallised in her mind, profoundly revolutionary given the fatalism of the day towards the collateral damage caused by hospitalisation: 'It may seem a strange principle to enunciate as a first requirement in a hospital that it should do the sick no harm.' This was as revolutionary as saying today 'the first requirement of military action is that it should do civilians no harm.' Of course, it has to be on the list somewhere, it could be the fourth or fifth requirement, but the *first*?

Six weeks later, in another letter to McNeill on the eve of her thirty-seventh birthday, bad food was no longer in the frame. She threw overboard the corpse of her original argument and directly contradicted the claim she had made during the war that the death rate had fallen because the men were now being sent in time to be saved:

> If it is objected that the condition of the men sent down from the Crimea during the first winter was such that they could not have recovered under any circumstances, I answer that the Land Transport Corps sent us down men in exactly the same condition the second winter, and they did recover.

Our mortality from 'Diseases of the Stomach and Bowels' was at Scutari 23.6 per cent; in Crimea 18.3 per cent.

Why this fatal increase? The condition of the buildings at Scutari is sufficient answer. You will observe that we lost at Scutari nearly 25 per cent more than we did in the Crimea from this cause alone. And the disease was chiefly generated within the building itself. I would furnish the amplest details on this all-important subject to any one interested in it officially as I have already done to Her Majesty.

Farr's calculations showed that there had been a huge variation in the death rates between different hospitals. It caused Nightingale to revise her previous assessment of the relative merits of each one. For example, in June 1856 she had written that the hospital at Balaclava in the Crimea was the worst, and now she found that it had a far better survival rate than any of the hospitals at Scutari. She had been used to evaluating hospitals on their organisational efficiency, not their patient survival rates. It was a rule of thumb with early statisticians like Farr that if something varied widely from place to place, then it could be reduced to zero because it must be strongly influenced by local conditions. It was not therefore particularly relevant that Nightingale's hospital complex near Constantinople had the highest death rate. Farr was not interested in creating a 'league table' of the type we use today to rate hospitals. The variation showed that it was not just the 5,000 deaths at Scutari that could have been prevented by better hygiene in the hospitals, but all the deaths from sickness in all the hospitals – a total of over 16,000. If true, this was a triumphant vindication of Farr's theories on the importance of building hygiene, which the English medical establishment had rejected when he returned from Paris.

Nightingale, finally convinced, started to rewrite her confidential report to give much greater prominence to hospital hygiene than in the version that she had discussed with McNeill in April. By the end of May she was sending to the printers a new section with the title 'Causes of Disaster at Scutari'. Earlier drafts of the preface still exist and show that before this rewrite it simply reiterated many of the McNeill report's criticisms of the army's supply organisation. The final printed preface deals almost exclusively with the sanitation disaster in the hospitals. It refers the reader to an appendix where 'we shall see how much of the mortality was due in the Crimean case also to the frightful state of the General Hospitals at Scutari; how much it depended upon the number which each regiment was unfortunately enabled to send to these pest-houses.'

The Appendix contains an improved version of Tulloch's sickness and mortality table which covered the seven months preceding his visit to the East with Sir John McNeill in the spring of 1855. Tulloch had printed this table after the war was over, in his rebuttal of the Board of Generals' report. When it appeared in the Appendix of Nightingale's confidential report, however, Tulloch's table had acquired an extra column, headed 'Sent to Scutari'. This allows a comparison between the survival rates of patients kept in the Crimea and of those sent to Nightingale's hospitals. With this additional information, it is possible to calculate how a soldier's chances of survival were affected by his choice of hospital.

By showing results separately for each of several dozen regiments, Tulloch's improved table showed clearly that regiments sharing different degrees of hardship, whether trench duty or difficulties in provisioning, had very different death rates, but in all cases the rate increased when the regiment sent its sick to Nightingale's hospital. Obviously, some regimental medical officers preferred to send all their sick to other hospitals, for example at Balaclava. The choice of hospital was therefore independent of the patient's previous history, and modern statistical analysis of Farr's table does give some confirmation that the choice of hospital was random. This randomisation of choice of hospital was a godsend to Farr. It overcame the problem that had prevented him from proving his theory that bigger London hospitals had higher death rates. Like many of Nightingale's associates, he had found the army a perfect laboratory for proving his social theories.

Nightingale now announced that Sutherland's Sanitary Commission should be given the credit for saving the army that she had previously given to McNeill's Supplies Commission. The death rate had dropped off dramatically when Sutherland had begun work. She did not like to hear of other possible contributing factors to this decline such as improved weather, better supplies, or less overcrowding in the hospitals. As before, but with a different objective, it was the political agenda that engaged her attention more than the facts. McNeill's political objective – reform of the army to limit hereditary aristocratic control – had shrunk in her eyes, and anyway by now McNeill had been vindicated and rewarded. In place of the handsome McNeill, honoured diplomat, friend and confidant of the Prime Minister, son of the Laird of Colonsay and raised in that island's idyllic environment, she now had William Farr for tutor. An unrecognised genius born out of the muck of a West Country hovel, whose cramped frame advertised the poverty of his youth; an unheeded prophet who told her of a conspiracy between landlords, the medical profession, and opponents of reform to keep Britain's poor in fatal squalor. Farr told her that she now had in her hands, and could publish in her report, irrefutable proof that expenditure on ventilation, flushed sewers, and fresh water could eliminate the horrific mortality from epidemic disease that was scourging the poor and decimating the nation's urban population every year.

Farr had opened up a new political landscape in front of Nightingale. This was no longer about saving the British Army. This was about saving Britain.

CHAPTER SIX

Cover-Up

The Royal Commission into the health of the Army sat from May to July 1857 in London, taking written and verbal evidence from a wide range of military and civilian experts, most of whom had spent time in the Crimea. Nightingale spent most of these three months trying to make the commission focus on the only subject that now interested her: building sanitation. Other subjects which she had fought successfully to include in the scope of the commission's enquiry, like army food rations, hospital supplies, and the training of doctors, seemed to her irrelevant now that with Farr's help she had identified 'the true causes of our disaster in the East.' She had completed the draft of her confidential report to focus on conditions inside the hospitals. She submitted this report to the commission as her evidence, so that it would be published instead of remaining a confidential report to the government. In it, she used the higher mortality in her own hospital to show that hygiene was far more important than medical care or hospital organisation.

The commission's President, Sidney Herbert, was reluctant to publish these revelations that were bound to trigger a new round of recriminations between politicians and officials, not to mention starting a controversy surrounding his government's dismissal of the sanitary reformer Edwin Chadwick just when he was most needed. Herbert had good reason for trying to stop the commission becoming yet another denunciation of official incompetence, because the blunders had occurred while he was responsible for the hospitals. He was also defensive about his former government's policies, making excuses for the failings of Lord Raglan, their army commander in the Crimea, before the Royal Commission as he had done before the House of Commons' Sebastopol Committee. Nightingale put pressure on Herbert as a friend, appealing to his sense of justice. They had known each other well for a decade, having been drawn together by their common interest in philanthropy. It was Herbert, of course, who as a Cabinet Minister had the idea of sending Nightingale to the East with a party of nurses.

At first she wanted Herbert to assign blame for the disaster to the medical staff whose incompetence in failing to see why the men were dying had caused the tragedy. Her desire to identify the guilty doctors who had misled her was new. When she first returned to England she often said that the system was to blame rather than individuals, and that if she reported on the hospitals of the East she would avoid 'all personal assaults upon individual Doctors whose conduct is only the result, to themselves, of the System under which they live'. But that was before she discovered the true cause of the disaster and her involvement in it. Now she wanted to identify the guilty parties. Her first choice as the person to blame for the disaster at Scutari was Sir John Hall, the Principal Medical Officer with the army in the East. 'I would only recall to your memory, the long series of proofs of his incredible apathy – beginning with the fatal letter approving of Scutari, October '54,' she wrote.

This allegation that Hall had given written approval of the Scutari buildings in October 1854 was not Nightingale's only charge against him. As the winter set in and the camps and hospitals of the static army became fouled with corpses and excrement, Hall and his staff did nothing about it, or so she claimed. Hall in response maintained that he and his staff had recommended the cleaning of the camps to their superiors who had ignored their advice. According to Hall, the civilian Sanitary Commission sent out by the new Palmerston Government only succeeded because they had power to act independently of the army, which he did not. In particular, he and his senior subordinate Mouat, who happens to be the most senior medical figure in the Crimea to have publicly defended Hall over the latter's widely criticised advice to his subordinates not to anaesthetise soldiers during amputations, claimed that they had warned about defective sanitation at Scutari.

Nightingale demanded that Herbert cross-examine Hall and Mouat to establish whether they had complained about the sanitation and if so to whom:

> I have thought a good deal of what you told me yesterday [she wrote to Herbert] and my conclusion is to make you a confidential Report great as is my objection to that system. If I were you I would say to Dr Mouat and Co. that you must have documentary evidence of what they state. Their object is [not to give this but] that you should make a general statement in the House of Commons. I know as a fact that none of these men knew what the others were doing. Therefore Mouat's statement can only be taken for himself. Nor would I take it even for himself without *documentary evidence*. But if Sir John Hall and Dr Mouat can prove that they did during the winter 54/55 make all the sanitary recommendations subsequently made by the Sanitary Commission, you will have done

immense good by bringing this out more even than by the other. For you will have fixed the responsibility in the right quarter for the operative causes which occasioned the loss of an army. You will have proved that if the Medical Officers had the knowledge they had not the power.

I trust that you will not let it drop. For I look upon the sanitary question as even more essential to the life of our army if possible than that of supplies.

This note shows that Herbert had been reluctant to cross-examine the senior army doctors for the public record about their claim that they had recommended sanitary improvements. Nightingale wanted him to do so because, if the cross-examination showed that they *did* make recommendations as they claimed, it would clearly place the blame on those to whom they made them. But during his cross-examination of Hall and Mouat, Herbert stayed away from the subject of whether these doctors had approved the sanitation in hospital buildings. Herbert asked Hall whether he had complained to the now dead Commander-in-Chief, Lord Raglan, about the unhealthy choice of campsites and about the inadequate rations. These were tactical matters that Raglan was responsible for, not the government far away in London. Hall replied that he had done so, and Herbert asked him to hand in documentary evidence, as Nightingale had suggested. But he did not ask Hall whether he had approved the defective hospitals at Scutari, as Nightingale had insisted he should. When Herbert called Mouat, Hall's subordinate, as a witness, neither Herbert nor Mouat raised the question of whether Mouat had complained about sanitation during the Crimean War. Herbert gave Mouat the opportunity to raise the subject by asking him whether he had ever complained about army sanitation. In reply, Mouat gave numerous examples of his tussles with the army over barracks hygiene in India and Ireland, but never mentioned the Crimea, and Herbert did not ask him about it.

Hall and Mouat did not therefore repeat their private allegations in front of the Royal Commission where they would have appeared in the published evidence. The case of Mouat, who according to Nightingale had asked Herbert to state in parliament that the doctors had made sanitary recommendations in the Crimea, is particularly striking. If Mouat did have the documentary evidence that Nightingale insisted that he should be made to produce, it has never seen the light of day. Nightingale did not have a high opinion of Mouat, judging from the bad character reference she gave him later when he was being considered for promotion: 'Mouat was the typical clever fellow, the unscrupulous blackguard, the unmitigated rogue. I believe I need hardly say that, in all this, I am referring exclusively to his conduct to his men, as *Inspecting* [i.e. Senior] Medical Officer. I do not refer at all to his medical practice, on which it is not my business to give an opinion.'

Nightingale's bad reference did not stop Mouat from rising to the top of the Army Medical Department, covered with honours of which the most prestigious was the Victoria Cross. It was given to him for bravery at the Charge of the Light Brigade. The problem for Mouat's reputation is that military historians do not see how he could have earned the VC during the Charge. He was supposed to have bravely treated a wounded officer on the battlefield, and drawn his sword to defend himself from Cossacks while doing so. But the wounded officer concerned had made his way back up the valley and fallen out of range of the Russian guns and under the noses of the English heavy cavalry. Military historians do not understand how Mouat could have been under fire nor how he could have been attacked by Cossacks. They have also been puzzled by the timing of Mouat's award, four years after the battle and after two other medical officers had received the Victoria Cross for more recent acts of bravery. Mouat's award came shortly after Herbert published Mouat's evidence to Nightingale's Royal Commission, in which Mouat avoided publicly repeating his allegations that would have reflected badly on Herbert and his government. His superior Dr Hall did pointedly drop a hint in his own evidence to the effect that there had not been enough medals for medical officers, and that Mouat had been under fire. Mouat himself had complained that medical officers at Nightingale's hospitals at Scutari were able to 'enjoy themselves in four-poster beds', while medical officers like him in the Crimea ran more risks and should therefore get more medals than those who worked with Nightingale. The problem of explaining the belated award of a VC to Mouat is, according to Mark Adkin, the historian of the Charge who was unaware of Mouat's role in Nightingale's Royal Commission, 'an interesting puzzle that will probably never be resolved.' The puzzle may have been resolved now that it has been shown that the reward came after Mouat did not produce his evidence against Herbert as Nightingale insisted that he should.

Another notable silence was that of Queen Victoria. According to her letter to McNeill, Nightingale's fight to publicise Farr's conclusions had already begun in the most unlikely quarter: the Royal Household: 'I will furnish amplest details . . . as I have already done to Her Majesty.' She can only be talking about a communication with Her Majesty between the end of March and the middle of May 1857. No trace of correspondence between Nightingale and Queen Victoria's household from this period exists in the Royal Archives, so we do not know what she told the Queen. But however her plea was made, it seems that it fell on deaf ears. From this time onwards, Nightingale seldom had a polite word to say about Queen Victoria. The following year she referred to herself as 'the greatest sufferer from the Queen's neglect, whose life would in fact have been saved, had she spoken the one word she could and ought to have spoken'.

Mouat, unmitigated rogue or not, may well have complained about the sanitation. But to Nightingale the question very quickly became irrelevant. Half way through the commission's proceedings, she became convinced that army doctors had no official training or responsibility in such matters and therefore could not be blamed for her disaster. She altered her confidential report to show that doctors could never be properly trained to approve the sanitary state of buildings, and that other experts would be necessary for this. We know of this change through her correspondence with Lord Grey, a former Secretary at War who had himself conducted a Royal Commission into the Administration of the Army twenty years before, to whom she sent an early draft of her confidential report for comments.

Lord Grey sent back a long review of her first draft in which he rejected her idea of removing the responsibility for preventive medicine from the Army Medical Department. Nightingale took account of his criticism by modifying her recommendations to demand only separate responsibility for building sanitation, and she tried to educate Sidney Herbert and the commission on this new distinction: 'Dear Mr Herbert,' she wrote on 1 July, 'I have had a long letter from Lord Grey on Army Hygiene matters which I want to show you. He is wrong in some matters. And the distinction between personal hygiene and that of buildings is not seen by him, nor indeed by your Commission. These will require two separate organisations being quite distinct in themselves.' The note probably did not improve Herbert's understanding of the distinction she was trying to draw. The mistake she made was to use the word hygiene in two contexts, making the distinction between personal hygiene and that of buildings appear to be only a question of object not one of technique. Elsewhere, she defined 'personal hygiene' to mean 'clothing, diet, duties, positions etc. of troops', and these had nothing to do with her new concept of building hygiene. She would have done better to use a different term for the cleanliness of buildings, but unfortunately the English language did not yet have such a term. 'Hygiene', 'sanitary,' and 'sanitation' to all but a few meant health care at that time – Hygeia was the Greek goddess of health, not of cleanliness. In his 1842 report on the *Sanitary Conditions of the Labouring Population*, Edwin Chadwick had investigated all aspects of health, and his proposed 'sanitary reforms' involved introducing the concept of environmental cleanliness into what was previously known as 'sanitary science', a science that at that time did not include environmental cleanliness, hence the need for reform. As a result of his efforts, 'sanitary reform' came to mean cleanliness, resulting in an almost complete reversal of the meaning of this term over the period 1842-1860. 'Sanitary' started out meaning health care devoid of environmental cleanliness, and ended up meaning environmental cleanliness alone. This has confused historians no end, as it confused Nightingale's Royal Commission.

But Nightingale was now clear in her own mind that Hall was no longer the main suspect in the case. As her understanding of the limitations of medical training and responsibility improved, she was able to identify another one. If doctors were not qualified to judge the sanitation of buildings, then who had ordered them to do so? If, despite their lack of formal training, they *had* alerted their superiors to the sanitary defects, then who was the superior who had the power to act and had failed to act? Either way, whether the doctors had complained about the sanitation or not, the trail must lead in the same direction. It led to the Cabinet Minister who had been responsible for the choice of the Scutari building as a hospital, or who had delegated this choice to an unqualified soldier and doctor (Lord Raglan and Dr John Hall). The trail led to a man whose sincerity and dedication to duty were recognised by all; a man who was admired by his colleagues of all political parties and was widely tipped as a future Prime Minister of England. He had been a member of the Cabinet at the time that the Scutari hospital was opened. He had volunteered to take temporary responsibility for the hospitals out of a personal interest in the subject, to help his colleague the Minister for War. He was, Nightingale now concluded, personally responsible for the loss of an army in those same lethal hospitals. He was her intimate friend Sidney Herbert, who was now the President of her Royal Commission.

By our standards it was not his fault. But Nightingale was a harsh judge, and part of her outrage was due to her discovery that England was being ruled by people who were not familiar with modern science and who made no attempt to consult those like William Farr who were. Herbert was a perfect example of this type of politician. To him, good intentions, good breeding, and a social conscience were the essential qualifications for a role in government. Herbert's biographer Lord Stanmore was a privileged observer as well as an equally ingenuous participant in the system of aristocratic rule that brought Sidney Herbert into government, and his memoir of Herbert is all the more revealing because of its author's uncritical acceptance of the system. The biographer himself was a part of this system; he was the son of Lord Aberdeen whose government had resigned in the face of parliamentary criticism of its handling of the war. Herbert had been a Minister in Aberdeen's government, and his biographer Lord Stanmore was at the time both an MP and his father's parliamentary secretary.

According to Lord Stanmore's account, Herbert's own education while at Oxford University had been limited: 'Sidney Herbert had originally intended to take honours, and had read for them; but he was induced, as his University course drew on, to desist from their pursuit, and took an ordinary degree in 1832. His health was at no time of his life strong, and it proved unequal to the strain imposed on it by severe study.'

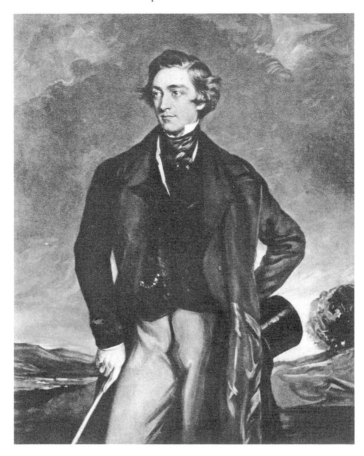

Sidney Herbert.

Herbert was the second son of Lord Pembroke. His older brother, Lord Herbert, had contracted an unwise marriage with a Sicilian lady and lived abroad. Sidney became wealthy himself as a result of a bequest of large estates in Shropshire and Ireland. He made a financial arrangement with his absent brother under which Sidney became the master of the ancestral home at Wilton, one of the finest in England. As a young man, Sidney Herbert was renowned for his charming manners and his physical grace. It was for these qualities, in addition to his aristocratic birth, that he was regarded as a potential ruler of the nation even while he was still at Oxford. Stanmore quotes from 'a periodical of the day' which interviewed Herbert in his rooms at Oriel College and, with a sarcasm so polished that it seems to have been lost on Lord Stanmore, recorded how little the future ruler was aware of modern approaches to government: 'Sidney Herbert's features and complexion are almost of feminine delicacy, and he is tall and slender almost to fragility ... We ask of his studies, as one who almost of necessity must bear a part, more or less influential, in the public affairs of this great commercial country. He points to Herodotus, to the Nichomachean ethics, and smilingly to Mr Newman's earliest sermons, and to a new edition of Wordsworth, Adam Smith and James Watt, trade, colonies, and commerce, have no place in that room.'

When Herbert first became a Cabinet Minister at the age of thirty-five, the political diarist Greville was dismissive: 'Sidney Herbert and Lord Lincoln come into the Cabinet . . . Sidney Herbert is a smart young fellow, but I remember no instance of two men who had distinguished themselves so little in Parliament being made Cabinet Ministers.' Three years later, Greville was even more dismissive: 'Lincoln has turned out worth a dozen Sidney Herberts.' The latter was the man whom everybody agreed would one day be Prime Minister of England. His suitability for this post lay in his ability to fit into any of the coalitions which were common at that time, because he had no enemies and no preconceived ideas or ideology other than a social conscience. A well known contemporary description of him has been widely misunderstood in this context. 'He was just the man to rule England. Birth, wealth, grace, tact, and not too much principle.' Some have interpreted the last words to mean 'unprincipled', but this is almost the exact opposite of what the speaker intended. The comment was a genuine compliment, reflecting on Herbert's open-mindedness. Nobody who knew him could possibly have called him unprincipled. He had no enemies, it may be true, but there were those who were envious. The man had too much. In addition to 'birth, wealth, grace, tact' there was one of the most magnificent stately homes in England and a ravishingly beautiful wife who was besotted with him. And what had he ever done to deserve any of it?

There is some of this envy, surely, in the comment made by an acquaintance of Herbert when Herbert's health began visibly to fail. 'How can a man like you get so ill? If I could lead your life I would live 1000 years, and never have a headache.' This was a remark of awful cruelty, because Herbert's protracted and fatal illness must have manifested itself within days of Nightingale telling him that she now held him personally responsible for the death of 16,000 men. Within a very short time she would find another whom she held even more responsible, but that could not absolve Herbert. The spark of life within him had died, though he worked on like an automaton for four more years.

Nightingale's obsession with tracking down those responsible for losing the first army sent to the East in 1854 was a product of the times as much as a personal challenge. Armies had been lost before, usually from the same causes, but the social and economic cost of such a calamity had recently escalated as a result of changes in society which the military authorities had not noticed. Nightingale, in the confidential report she was writing for the Cabinet, exhumed the old reports from the Peninsular War and showed that troops who were billeted indoors in comfort died in great numbers while those who shivered beneath the stars usually lived. There had been no attempt at the time to find out why.

What had changed was that by 1854 the army was no longer made up of 'the scum of the earth, enlisted for drink' as the Duke of Wellington is reputed to have said with memorable objectivity fifty years before. At the time Wellington made that remark, men enlisted for at least twenty years, and the army was a dumping ground for those who had no hope of gainful employment. By the 1850s, such people had become rarer, and a new form of enlistment – Limited Service Enlistment – made the army an attractive opportunity for young men temporarily at a loose end and wishing to see a bit of the world. The main opponent of the Limited Service Act in parliament had been none other than Sidney Herbert.

The men who died in their thousands on the floors of the eastern hospitals were therefore a loss to the economy of Victorian England in a way that earlier generations of soldiers had not been. One of Nightingale's nurses described a typical one of them: 'Charles was a lad pretty well educated, the son of a Berwickshire farmer who died before his children were settled in life or provided for. He went to London to seek employment; failing to find it he wrote home saying that rather than hang about idle, or return to be a burden on his mother, he would enlist as a private.' He died at Scutari in February 1855. Such men were part of the mobile labour force of the new industrial economy, and the country felt the loss even more sharply than the sum of individual bereavements. It was this communal loss that Nightingale tried to represent when she spoke of 'my 18,000 children'.

Nightingale wanted the country to know why so many young men had died. She wanted the country to know that they had been guinea-pigs in one of the most perfect imaginable experiments, the results of which proved that Farr, Chadwick, and the 'sanitarians', as they were becoming known, were right. The reason for early mortality in all walks of life was defective building cleanliness. Her confidential report, nearing completion, used the results of the dreadful experiment at Scutari to prove this. She wanted Sidney Herbert to accept this report as her written evidence before the Royal Commission, and print it in full in the commission's public report.

Her confidential report, entitled *Notes on Matters affecting the Health, Efficiency, and Hospital Administration of the British Army, Founded Chiefly on the Experience of the late War* was being privately printed for submission to the government during July 1857 as the Royal Commission heard its final witnesses. Nightingale was overwhelmed by stress and paper-work, and had acquired a rather unusual part-time secretary: Arthur Clough, her cousin's husband, a young man whose early brilliance had led disappointingly to a number of complicated poems and a clerical job in the Civil Service. Clough was in the Lake District during July, exchanging proofs of her confidential report with Nightingale and her printers. He wrote to her in mid-July telling her that he could complete the printing in time for the Cabinet to authorise its release to the Royal Commission as her evidence.

But Herbert, the commission's President, did not want to publish her data on the higher mortality at Scutari. He thought that if hospital cleanliness was the key lesson to be learned, she should limit her evidence to the subject of future hospital construction. For safety's sake, he wanted her to submit written answers to agreed written questions. She wrote to him rejecting this proposal:

> Dear Mr Herbert, I have really tried to write questions for my own examination as you directed and I cannot. I feel thus:
> 1. I am quite as well aware as you can be that it is inexpedient and even unprincipled to go back into past delinquencies.
> 2. What is more, I feel for you who were victimised by a System, which you could not possibly understand, till you saw its results.
> 3. But it would be equally untrue and unconscientious for me to give evidence upon an indifferent matter like that of hospital construction and leave untouched the great matters which will affect the mortality of our sick (and have affected them) far more than any architectural plan could do.

Nightingale wrote an almost identical letter to Sir John McNeill in which she referred to the unnamed accused person as 'he . . . victimised by a system . . .', showing that she was accusing Herbert himself and not his government collectively. She went on to explain to Herbert why she could not keep quiet: 'People, Government, and Sovereign all think that these matters have been remedied while I think that nothing has been done. It would be treachery to the memory of my dead if I were to allow myself to be examined on a mere scheme of hospital construction.' She added that she wanted her confidential report to be published, otherwise the government would be free to ignore the inconvenient parts of it. Finally, she threatened to boycott the commission if Herbert refused to let her tell the whole truth: 'The only question is: what can be done to prevent a recurrence of the evils from which we have suffered? And I ought not to consent to be examined on anything less – though I would much rather not be examined at all.'

The Royal Commission did not print her confidential report as evidence in their public report. Of course, they could not have done so unless and until the War Minister agreed to remove its confidential status. Perhaps he had originally intended to do so; perhaps the Cabinet had requested it as a hedge against failure to secure a Royal Commission. But it seems unlikely that Lord Panmure could have foreseen that Nightingale would turn her confidential report into such a deadly missile. He must have been awestruck at the sight of the missile heading towards its chosen target – his long-time political rival Sidney Herbert and the previous government in which Herbert had served. But the aristocracy closed ranks – their collective position was too precarious – and he refused to let it be published.

Her report containing the secret of Scutari has never been published, though twelve months after she completed it she sent copies to a number of distinguished people, each time with a covering letter containing strict instructions not to let anyone else see it or even to leave it lying around. After the deaths of the recipients, these copies found their way into specialised libraries and created the false impression that it had been published after all.

Herbert may have argued that suppression of Nightingale's account of the disaster at Scutari was necessary to protect the new public enthusiasm for nursing which accompanied the adulation of Nightingale in the press, in ballads, pictures, memoirs, poetry, and works of fiction. With such a reputation working for her, he would have argued, there was no limit to the amount of good that Nightingale could do towards her old ambition of opening up the nursing profession. To expose the dark side of her work at Scutari would not only cause unnecessary pain to the families of those who had died, but also destroy both Nightingale's reputation and the new freedom of educated women to seek respectable employment.

Nightingale now seemed to care little for the survival of hospital nursing as a profession. Scutari had convinced her that nursing improvements were of low priority. Facilitating female careers in nursing was a sub-optimisation that addressed the wrong part of the problem. Her most fiery and popular book *Notes on Nursing,* written soon afterwards, was in fact propaganda directed *against* doctors, hospitals, and hospital nursing. Her reputation as the merciful angel of Scutari was no longer an embarrassment to her, it was a devilishly cruel and macabre joke at her expense. The Nightingale Fund, which she held in trust for training hospital nurses, had become a monster that terrified her. She tried unsuccessfully to resign from the Fund and then turned her back on its Nightingale Training School.

The quarrel between Herbert and Nightingale over the suppression of the evidence was to have devastating results for both of them. Witnessing Nightingale's anguish may also have been too much for her secretary Arthur Clough, whose health went into rapid and fatal decline shortly afterwards. Clough was not a worshipper of Nightingale, but there must have been a strange affinity between them judging from his frequent use of intense water imagery in his poems. Running water is the bloodstream of any sanitary system, and Nightingale's later work on India revolved around securing water supplies. One of Clough's more simple and pessimistic poems, summarising his disillusion with the intellectual pursuits that had been his whole life, even seemed to equate futile intellectual effort with defective plumbing through its image of 'broken cisterns':

Away, haunt not thou me,
Thou vain philosophy!
Unto thy broken cisterns wherefore go,
When from the secret treasure-depths below,
Wisdom at once, and Power,
Are welling, bubbling forth, unseen, incessantly?
Why labour at the dull mechanic oar,
When the fresh breeze is blowing.
And the strong current flowing,
Right onward to the Eternal Shore?

An intimate exposure to Nightingale's problems in the summer of 1857 would certainly have weakened Clough's already enfeebled will to row his boat against the current.

Sidney Herbert must have made a compromise with Nightingale because eventually she agreed to give evidence to the Royal Commission that avoided blaming him or his former government. It seems that Herbert must have promised that he would devote his political reputation to her objectives if she agreed to limit her public evidence. She referred to some kind of obligation in a letter to McNeill a few months later: 'Sidney Herbert is the most sensitive of men on the subject of his personal obligations, this gives me a hold over him.'

The Royal Commission entirely suppressed Farr's comparative analysis of hospitals and Nightingale's discussion of it. In the commission's final report there was only one mention of the excess deaths at Scutari compared to other hospitals. That was in a quite irrelevant written response to a question asking Nightingale how she would organise a general hospital. Quoting a statement from Sir John Hall that among 442 patients treated at Balaclava hospital the death rate was twelve per month, she wrote: 'If these men had been sent to Scutari, there would have died not twelve but 189.' Herbert reviewed her written evidence before allowing it into the report, and allowed this fragmentary comparison because it had already been published by Sutherland in an exchange of pamphlets with Sir John Hall when the latter tried to discredit Sutherland's report of his earlier Sanitary Commission. In any case, as a single comparison between two hospitals, without any justification, it did not give much away.

Nor did the army's official *Medical and Surgical History of the British Army*, published in the following year, support Nightingale's allegation of higher mortality at Scutari. The numbers of patients sent by each regiment to Scutari, which convinced Tulloch and Nightingale that her hospitals at Scutari had a higher death rate, have never appeared in any published document and have not, as far as is known, been preserved in any official archive. If Nightingale had not given copies of her confidential report to individuals whom she could trust to preserve it for posterity, we would never have known about the secret of Scutari.

Instead of analysing the medical errors of the Crimean War, the Royal Commission's final report dwelt more on the continuing high mortality among soldiers in barracks in peacetime. This was in line with Herbert's plan to focus more on opportunities for future improvement than on the mistakes of the past. It was known that mortality among soldiers in peacetime was higher than among civilians; there was no agreement on how to account for it. Various explanations were possible including immoral behaviour, alcohol, smoking, and idleness. It was only when they discovered the real cause of the huge mortality at Scutari that Farr and Nightingale could argue convincingly that the same cause – bad sanitation in the crowded barracks – accounted for the high peacetime mortality.

The commissioners' report affirmed that bad sanitation was causing unnecessary deaths in barracks in peacetime. But it did not quote the results of the 'Scutari experiment' to justify this conclusion, even though it was the strongest possible evidence. Instead, the commission relied on the less convincing evidence that most of the deaths in peacetime were due to respiratory diseases. The commissioners discussed the mortality at Nightingale's hospital at Scutari not by comparing it to that at other hospitals, but by comparing it 'before and after' sanitary improvements were made, using the difference to push for similar improvements in barracks.

Herbert did agree to include in the report a diagram that Nightingale had produced with Dr Farr's help to illustrate the high mortality from sickness. This diagram was carefully constructed to convey only the main 'before and after sanitary improvements' message. It consists of two polygons, one swollen with preventable deaths covering the first year of the war, and the other much smaller covering the period after the Sanitary Commission did its work. Farr sent several variations of the diagrams to Herbert with the comment: 'Miss Nightingale kindly promises to place these diagrams in your hands. They throw a terrible light on the seat of her labours – which surpasses all I had imagined. I suspect that a Defoe could scarcely bring it home to our minds.' Afterwards Farr enjoyed a long professional relationship with Nightingale during which both of them were perpetually in hot water with the medical establishment for their criticism of hospitals. Farr's finest hour came when he managed to coax his most advanced life table – the English Life Table No. 3 – out of one of the very few working machines ever to be built using the principles of Thomas Babbage's Difference Engine. He thus became the first person to calculate and print a table of numbers with a computer, to meet demand from the life insurance industry.

Farr later may have had reason to regret that Nightingale's confidential report was suppressed, and specifically that she thwarted an attempt to publish it in America. 'Had the conclusions which Florence Nightingale reached been heeded in the Civil War in America, hundreds of thousands of lives might have been saved,' wrote one expert many years later when referring to the confidential report. One of Farr's sons ran away to America and joined the Union Army in the Civil War. He fought at Gettysburg but then wrote to his father asking for his help in getting out. Not being particularly well-connected, Farr tried to enlist the help of medical colleagues in America, to no avail. The boy died in the closing days of the war of fever caught in an army hospital.

The events immediately following the censoring of Nightingale's evidence to the Royal Commission are not well documented. The archive material is much sparser and does not allow us to follow her evolving thought as it does during her gradual discovery of the causes of Crimean mortality. The nature of the compromise she reached with Herbert can only be guessed at in the light of subsequent events. For example, she may have agreed never to allow her findings to be published, but in terms that did not prevent her from privately circulating it after a period of twelve months had elapsed. Just as she initially blamed Hall and then moved on to blame Herbert when the limits of Hall's responsibility became apparent to her, so she may have decided that the trail did not stop at Herbert. Without any written evidence all that can be said is that much of what came later can be explained by her discovery of another guilty party. It may even be that Herbert defended himself by casting blame on this other person. It might not have been very chivalrous, but he might with some justification have told Nightingale that he had done everything that was necessary to ensure the success of his hospital plan.

He had, after all, selected an expert to implement his ill-thought-out vision of a general hospital remote from the battlefields. A person who was to be present on the spot, equipped with a regional intelligence network covering all the hospitals in the war zone, and who reported directly to the Cabinet in London. A person who was one of the world's recognised experts in hospital management, not just an impractical philanthropist. In charge, trained for the job, and equipped with unprecedented powers, there was one person who could have made the whole Scutari experiment a success. This person, she might easily have concluded, could have saved an army. This person, of course, was Florence Nightingale.

Nightingale referred, in a letter to McNeill, to 'the manslaughter committed in 1854'. She was still blaming the failure to feed the troops at the front, not yet having met Farr and become convinced that the disease was generated inside the hospital. Does her later discovery make her an accessory to manslaughter? One can only answer this question on the evidence, and the evidence points clearly to *not guilty*. Unless she in some way obstructed or opposed remedial sanitary construction, her ignorance of the cause of death was not culpable. The new War Minister, receiving her assertion that the previous high death rate had been due only to the poor state of the patients on arrival, knew that she was unqualified to make that judgment, and he was not influenced by it.

But, if she *felt* guilty, and there is evidence that she did, could this prove that some evidence has been destroyed that would have convicted her? No it doesn't because, as her lost diaries show, she was unusually susceptible to social guilt. She considered herself guilty by being born into the wealthiest of the wealthy classes: 'In London there have been the usual amount of Charity Balls, Charity Concerts, Charity Bazaars, whereby people bamboozle their consciences and shut their eyes . . . England is surely the country where luxury has reached its height and poverty its depth.'

Her fortune or her misfortune was that she had volunteered to be a leader, perhaps not realising how natural it is for male leaders to shrug off their mistakes. The French *Grande Armée* that marched into Russia in 1812 lost 300,000 men even before arriving at Borodino, the first big battle, the vast majority of them from disease. We don't see Napoleon moping about this preventable loss of two thirds of his army. It's easier for men to be leaders: they're only in it for the glory, but Nightingale had been conscience-stricken all her life about the mistreatment of those on the lowest level of society, and she could not help taking this disaster personally.

It is unlikely that she would have blamed herself for not knowing that building hygiene was necessary to health. Few people held this belief at the time, and she had little experience of such things before the war. There is no evidence of a mania for environmental cleanliness before she met Farr. A review of Nightingale's letters home from Scutari when the epidemic was at its peak shows that her endless and justified complaints and requests for action included no comment on any need for improvements in ventilation or drainage there. But there was no reason why she should associate these matters with the symptoms that she observed; neither did she have any training or experience that would cause her to question the doctors' claim that the men were already dying when they entered the hospital.

Her expansion of the Barrack Hospital was not necessarily a bad thing. It may have reduced the overcrowding and the mortality. But could she have made the workmen drill holes in the roof as well, as the Sanitary Commission later did? She kept her own window open because of the smell, but the windows in the wards did not open. Sutherland's Sanitary Commission smashed 400 panes of glass with their own hands on their second day at Scutari. Could she have done this? Yes, judging by her other building work it was within the limits of her power, but she had no experience with which to justify it to her colleagues.

She had also put pressure on Lord Raglan to send more patients to Scutari instead of leaving them in primitive hospitals at the front where, as she later found out, more of them would have lived. She applied this pressure by opposing his requests for nurses to be sent to the other general hospitals. When she was overruled and the nurses did go, she called it 'a mistake' and refused to supervise them, as we have seen in the account by Mrs Davis. This was a part of her plan to centralise the hospitals and the nursing service, and reflected her desire to bring more patients under her undeniably superior standard of nursing care. But it was a sub-optimisation, because her superior nursing could not make up for the worse state of her hospital. When Raglan decided in May 1855 to stop sending patients to her, she was upset. It is unlikely that she would later consider this to be a major contributor to the disaster because her protests did not, after all, stop the nurses from leaving.

Her wartime failure to exploit the energy and drive of the maverick nurses who deserted to the front – some of them immoral, intemperate, and even possibly insane – as part of a distributed system of hospital control was one of the missed opportunities during the war. It was another lesson that she was to put to great use later. The most obvious use that she could have made of the nurses in the outposts was in the collection of information, for example mortality statistics that after a few weeks would have revealed why and where the men were dying. Her later obsession with mortality statistics shows that this omission must have tormented her, but she never tried to hide the evidence of her failure to share information. In several documents that she preserved (including the notes of her first visit to Farr's General Registry Office quoted earlier) she bemoaned the absence of army mortality statistics when in fact they existed all the time! As she found out later, Colonel Tulloch collected a comprehensive set of them covering the months when the tragedy was occurring under her nose, and it was these statistics that later allowed Farr to diagnose the cause.

Colonel Tulloch got his statistics from the army in the field simply by asking. He admits that he had no authority to ask for such information, as he was supposed to be investigating the supplies, but he was a seasoned sleuth and realised that he could exploit the desire of one part of the organisation to expose the inadequacies of another part. The doctors were claiming that the army was creating too much work for them by treating the soldiers too harshly, and they were prepared to give him what they thought was evidence of this: 'At a very early stage of our enquiry,' wrote Tulloch, 'we saw the necessity, before venturing on any report as to the suffering of the troops from the non-distribution of the supplies, that the extent of the sickness and the mortality during the previous winter should be carefully examined. It is true we had no authority for this extension of our enquiries, but it appeared absolutely requisite to test the allegations against the army officers by numerical evidence. The medical officers supplied the information readily, as affording one of the best evidences of their unparalleled exertions, and of the difficulties they had to contend with.' These medical statistics had been regularly kept at regimental level since before Nightingale's arrival, and if she had used the same method of enquiry she could have discovered them in time to act immediately.

Worse, Tulloch makes it clear that it was the failure of Nightingale's Scutari hospital to send mortality statistics to Nightingale's nominal superior in the Crimea that prevented the authorities at that end from discovering that they were shipping men off to almost certain death. Nightingale read the following observation by Tulloch shortly after she met Farr:

> It is one of the most serious considerations connected with the history of this period that the loss by disease was at first much underestimated. For several months, no accurate or complete returns appear to have been received from Scutari, to show what had become of the invalids sent there. It was only by degrees that the small proportion who returned, of those who had left the Crimea sick, awakened a suspicion of the fatal character of the diseases, and of the extent to which the constitution of the troops had suffered by the hardships and privations they had undergone. Had it even been surmised by the principal medical and military authorities that the loss in that army averaged about a battalion every week by disease alone, measures would have been adopted to check it.

Tulloch meant by this that if the staff at Scutari had informed their superiors in the Crimea of the death rate at Scutari, the authorities would have stopped the flow of patients one way or another. This did happen, eventually, and is partly responsible for the fall in mortality as Nightingale discovered after the war. At the time when the Sanitary Commission was arriving, the correspondent of *The Times* was writing from the front: 'It is strange we have got up so few convalescents from Scutari. The hospitals there seem to swallow up the sick forever.' The Coldstream Guards had to send a Colonel down to Scutari to see what had happened to the missing men, and when he reported back that they were all dead his regiment sent no more. He must have informed Dr Hall, the PMO in the Crimea, who claimed in a pamphlet after the war that two weeks before the Sanitary Commission arrived he had warned: 'the mortality from fever at Scutari is so great that I send men down with great reluctance.'

When criticising the failure of those at Scutari to send statistics to Hall, Tulloch probably had no intention of pointing the finger at Nightingale. It may not have been Nightingale's job to inform her superiors in the Crimea of the death rate. But then, neither does it seem to have been anyone else's job, and Nightingale was probably the only person in the hospital who didn't believe in this excuse for inaction. She *did* have the necessary statistical skills, because she had insisted on studying mathematics against the wishes of her family. Even before the war she had admired the work of the statistician Quetelet, and on her own initiative she had collected statistics from different hospitals throughout Europe. This one omission of hers would probably have been enough to convince her that she had been partly to blame for the disaster.

On a more emotional level, it must have occurred to her that she had been far too ready to listen to her charismatic hero Sir John McNeill, who told her that her patients in the winter were already dying. This didn't make any difference to the early mortality, but it had made her go out on a limb and promote his theory publicly and officially, which weakened her credibility after the war when she began to promote the opposite conclusion. Her sanitarian colleagues had to endure barbed comments about 'one who has become a recent convert to your cause', and she had written at least one letter which could now be used against her in which she had denied that her hospital was at fault. Regardless of whether there had been any impropriety with McNeill, it was clear that the woman who had slept with the key to the nurses' quarters under her pillow, and had forbidden her nurses to fraternise with the doctors and orderlies, had let her heart rule her head and had been blinded by an emotional attachment to a man. This must have increased her remorse.

Her father had made her a proud woman, and now her associates and her enemies could see the angel of Scutari publicly admitting that she had been wrong, and that the cause of the calamity was much closer to her and her sponsor Sidney Herbert than she had loudly claimed. It was a grotesque humiliation, particularly in front of her father and her sister. Her mother was less important; ignorant of what was going on, Fanny Nightingale had watched in awe as grandees like the Duke of Newcastle called at the Burlington Hotel to see her daughter. 'These men seem to make her opinions their law,' she wrote to her husband, unaware of how many great political reputations lay in the palm of her daughter's hand when she was obsessively tracking down those responsible for the martyrdom of the common soldier. It is not clear whether her mother ever found out the truth about Florence's humiliation by the findings of her own Royal Commission. But her father and sister were another matter. Parthe had crowed to the world during and after the war how holy and dedicated her sister was, but only a year before the war she derided Florence's hospital ambitions: 'I believe she has little or none of what is called charity or philanthropy,' wrote Parthe to a mutual friend. She went on:

> She is ambitious – very and would like to regenerate the world with a grand *coup de main* or some fine institution, which is a very different thing. Here she has a circle of admirers who cry up everything she

does or says as gospel. It is the intellectual part which interests her, not the manual. When she nursed me everything which intellect and kind intention could do was done but she was a shocking nurse. Whereas her influence on people's minds and her curiosity in getting into varieties of minds is insatiable, after she has got inside they generally cease to have any interest for her.

And now the sister who could write those terrible words was breathing down Florence's neck and learning her innermost secrets, despite Florence's desperate attempts to keep her away from London. Parthe had copied out the letter that Florence had written to McNeill when she had finally admitted to what had really killed her patients. Parthe must have understood the implications of her sister's discovery. Did she tell their father? He must have found out, one way or another. How could Florence bear to face him? The man who had raised her with infinite care to be something in the world, to compensate for his lack of worldly success. The man who was happy to live in her shadow, who had written to her so openly of his attempt to exploit her fame to get himself elected to parliament. That good man who had called her, with innocent and transparent pride, 'you, my only genius'.

All her life she had been trying to prove that her mother and sister were wrong; that she could create a secular female nursing profession. All her life she had been trying to impress her father, to reward him for the support he had given her against them. She had written to her parents late in the war: 'If my name and having done what I could for God and mankind has given you pleasure that is real pleasure to me. I shall love my name now. Life is sweet after all.' And, to her sister: 'I have done my duty. I have identified my fate with that of the heroic dead. It has been a great cause.'

It was a proud young woman who had written these words. It would be hard to find a more severe case of *hubris*. The final straw for her came when the government refused to publish her report with its convincing statistics showing that hospital conditions caused the high mortality, with which she now hoped to revive the campaign for building hygiene in Britain. She collapsed mentally and physically around 20 August 1857, three weeks after trying and failing to get her crucial evidence published by the Royal Commission in its closing days. There is a gap in the surviving family papers at this time, and no details survive of her collapse. Perhaps this is fortunate.

Usually the subject of a biography dies at the end of the book, but it is easier to make sense of Florence Nightingale by imagining that the woman we have been reading about died here, aged thirty-seven. A large part of her did die in the Burlington Hotel on that quiet August day, just after the Royal Commission had ended its frantic three months of activity,

Parliament had gone into recess, and the politicians had deserted London for their country estates.

There have been many problems trying to reconcile her statements and actions before and after her breakdown, usually leading to charges of 'inconsistency' against her. One of these so-called inconsistencies of the early post-Royal Commission period is her withering remark about doctors, made to Sidney Herbert in 1859: 'As for doctors civil and military there must be something in the smell of medicine which renders absolute administrative incapacity. And it must be something very strong for they all have an opportunity to develop administrative capacity, almost more than in any other profession.' If she had so little confidence in doctors, it has been said, why did she appoint four of them to positions on the Council of the Nightingale Fund in 1856? The answer is that she put them on the Council before she found out, during the Royal Commission, that doctors were a part of the problem.

When she first went to Scutari she had gone to extreme lengths to submit, at least in appearance, to the medical staff. She threatened her nurses with instant dismissal if they attended to a patient before being ordered to do so by the doctors. After 1857, there was a complete reversal of this: she insisted that army nurses must report not to the medical officers but direct to the Minister of War. For her this was non-negotiable. These 'inconsistencies' show that trying to use a biographical portrait of Nightingale up to 1857 as a guide to her later life is like trying to find your way around London using a 200-year old map. All the major inconsistencies in her life occur on either side of the August 1857 divide.

After that date, Nightingale seems to have suffered very badly from repressed feelings of guilt. This guilt was worse than the 'survivor syndrome', which diminishes the feelings of self-worth of someone who survives a major tragedy. It must have come from the feeling that her negligence and arrogance had contributed to the loss of the army, possibly compounded by a realisation that she had at first refused to admit to the truth and had then unwisely allowed a cover-up, thus betraying three times 'her murdered men'.

Although she destroyed many documents from this period, it is not likely that they would have contained any expression of guilt. She probably could not put her feelings into words, at least in the first decade or so. A failure to articulate such feelings would give them a tremendous power as a driving force in her life. What can't be talked about can only be – and must be – acted upon. Assuaging her guilt through work for the sanitarian cause and other social reforms became a full-time obsession. There could be no clearer indication of how her overwhelming workload helped her to suppress her guilt than a letter she wrote in 1869 about her struggle:

I say nothing of my immense Scutari Hospitals, because even now when I look back to what those slaughter houses were when we first came to them it seems to me like a horrid spectre one is afraid of conjuring up out of the dark corner of one's mind in which it must be ever present, ready to spring out upon one, if one were not so overwhelmed with present work.

Many different explanations for her collapse after the Royal Commission have been advanced over the years, and Nightingale's own explanation for it is itself revealing. She believed that the trigger for her breakdown was her family. Her mother and sister were persecuting her, following her to London, lodging in the same hotel, and pretending to help her with the Royal Commission while in fact obstructing her work. They had always obstructed her, had never loved her, and now they were trying to claim credit for making her famous. If they had only left her alone during the Royal Commission she 'could have waded through'. 'What have my mother and sister ever done for me? They like my glory, they like my pretty things. Is there anything else they like in me?' Most significant of all, it was her sister's ungrateful and spiteful behaviour that had caused 'the disease which is now bringing me to my grave.'

Any thirty-seven-year-old woman who has been running a vast nursing empire, has seen thousands of men die unnecessarily in front of her eyes, and has become a national heroine, would find it difficult to convince an impartial observer that the attitudes of her mother and sister, however neurotic, were sufficient to ruin her health and happiness. She was placing the entire blame for her situation on people whose only crime was their genetic closeness to her. They had created her, or were mirrors of her. Irrational hatred of those who are genetically closest appears to be consistent with displaced self-loathing.

This diagnosis that Nightingale suffered from repressed guilt explains some of her later writings and behaviour. First, she had a habit of omitting all references to the Crimean War whenever she – rarely – praised her own achievements. Second, she punished herself with what was virtually a sentence of life imprisonment beginning in the weeks after the end of the Royal Commission. 'Last month,' she wrote in September 1861, makes four years that I have been imprisoned by sickness.' Third, she further developed her religious beliefs to excuse the errors of philanthropists, holding that a well-intentioned mistake will always be turned to the benefit of mankind. And finally, as we shall see when we look at her working methods, she adopted a completely new leadership style, characterised by one over-riding feature: if she had used the same approach at Scutari, the disaster would never have happened. She was like a general who loses a battle and, realising with hindsight how he could have won it, spends the rest of his life trying to find an enemy with whom to fight the same battle over again to achieve the correct result.

On 21 August, she fled from London to the spa town of Malvern. On 25 August, she wrote a short note from Malvern to her family saying she was glad to be alone. When Dr Sutherland wrote to her telling her not to work too hard, a letter flew back bizarrely accusing him of being in league with her sister Parthe. Somehow she got control of herself again. The mental turmoil subsided as she began work at Malvern on the sequel to the Royal Commission – designing a number of committees with executive powers to reform army administration. Her condition stabilised.

The secret remedy was undoubtedly her spiritual beliefs. As she had said to Lord Raglan: 'My father's religious and social ethics make us strive to be the pioneers of the human race.' In particular, she formed the protective notion that what had happened to her was not a catastrophe but rather the first small step in God's grand plan for her. 'Mankind creating mankind' is a process that requires mistakes, comparable to the process of natural selection. Her use of this mental construction to convert her disaster into a consolation and a strength is an impressive testimony to the power of human thought. In her analysis, her God could not have been wrong to send an ignorant woman to Scutari. Sooner or later, someone with a sense of duty to Him would have to make the mistake if repetitions were to be stopped. It was not very hard for an imaginative young woman to come to this mystical conclusion, because there was something unearthly about the scale and design of her personal disaster that made it look like the result of a heavenly plan.

Everything had conspired to prevent her from avoiding the tragedy, and to maximise its impact upon her. She had been so close to recognising the epidemic for what it was. Only weeks before going to Scutari she had noted in a letter to her sister the new evidence that environmental factors were responsible for disease, and had castigated the Church of England for its futile prayers for deliverance from the cholera epidemic that was then terrorising London: 'You [the Church of England, with which Parthe was more aligned than Florence] pray against "plague, pestilence, and famine", when God has been saying more loudly every day this week that those who live ten feet above a pestilential river will die, and those who live forty feet above will live.'

Her vague notion that cholera was associated with dirty water did not have a scientific basis yet. She did not know that people who lived close to a river tended to get their drinking water from it instead of walking to a pump. Dr John Snow convinced himself (but no one else at the time) of the importance of drinking water just two weeks after she wrote those words by taking the handle off the contaminated Broad Street water pump and stopping the Soho cholera epidemic dead in its tracks. It may seem strange that the woman who held such relatively advanced views could have failed to see three months later that the filth in the unventilated Barrack Hospital was killing her patients by the thousand. But her experience in the London cholera epidemic was of no use to her because not many of the patients at Scutari died with the unmistakable symptoms of cholera.

Destiny also took unfair advantage of her at Scutari by sending her patients with symptoms ghastly enough to distract attention from anything they caught after arriving in her hospital. Many of them were starved and frost-bitten, so that it seemed a miracle that they were alive at all. Their limbs were blackened and mortified; some had lost their hands and feet to frost-bite and their bones protruded from their disintegrating extremities. Long-untended wounds were infested with maggots. It was easy to believe the doctors' view that they were already beyond recovery.

These sufferers whom she failed to rescue were the 'common soldier', an object of veneration to her when she was at Scutari and central to many philanthropists' ideas of social improvement. She was continually in trouble for spending too much time on this brute and not enough on their officers. One of the most hostile senior officers complained to the Commander-in-Chief that she habitually neglected her 'equals or superiors': 'Whatever philanthropy she may have on a great scale, she does not appear to be amiable in ordinary intercourse with her equals or superiors. She likes to *govern* and bestows all her tenderness upon those who *depend* upon her. For instance, she will not give a thought upon any *officer* who may be in the most wretched State.' This was, of course, an exaggeration, but there was a grain of truth in it.

'Bestows all her tenderness on those who *depend* on her' seems to have been a serious criticism in those days. In fact, her philosophy made her dependent on *them,* the common soldiers. Now she found that her fate had made her betray them over and over again. But it was even more meaningful than that, for these were not just *any* common soldiers. The men whom fate sent to her hospitals that winter in the last extremities of suffering were the very same common soldiers whose bravery and initiative had astonished the Russians during the victories of the war's earliest months. Acting largely without orders, they had overwhelmed a superior Russian position beside the River Alma. They had stood at Balaclava in what was to become famous as the 'Thin Red line', again without orders, and showed that British soldiers were the only infantry in the world who would not yield to cavalry when fighting in the open in line rather than in a square. They had pressed to participate in the Charge of the Light Brigade, accepting horrific losses and then routing ten times their number of Russian cavalry behind the guns. For maximum effect, these heroic common soldiers had to be consigned to indifferent and incompetent officers so that they could be reduced to living wreckage in the trenches and then sent to young Florence Nightingale in a pest-house, to teach her God's laws of hygiene.

No, you wouldn't have to be a religious fanatic to suspect that there had been some intelligence at work here, an intelligence which particularly wanted to make use of Florence Nightingale. Whatever faults she may have had, *her* God would not create this much evil just to punish her for a little bit of arrogance. Therefore it must be for a different purpose. And her friend Sidney Herbert, who had made as many omissions as she had, must also have been part of God's design. Without him, she would not have been sent there to be taught what she had to learn. 'Your mistakes', as she had remarked to her sister a few weeks before leaving for the war, 'are part of God's plan.'

This was what she came to believe at Malvern, during her solitary breakdown. This was how she managed to hide her feelings of guilt from herself. The education that her father had given her was as strong and at the same time as finely wrought as one of those elaborate early Victorian steam engines. The image that seems to fit her temporary breakdown best is that of a safety valve that, under the pressure of an unexpected load which prevents the piston moving, opens to release a rush of steam. Then it is as if she ruthlessly slams a steel wedge into the valve. From then on, we can only cringe and wait for the possible explosion as the engine strains silently against the load. Then, bearing testimony to her father's workmanship as an educator, the machinery begins to move.

She refused to allow anyone to come to Malvern to visit her but her father went anyway and forced his way into her room. They had a secret conversation. He was so shaken that he refused to talk about it with anyone at the time. Years later, when her mother insisted that her father explain what happened that week in Malvern, he reluctantly provided a few details. He described the scene in her room, which was on the top floor of the house used by a well-known hydropathic doctor, where she sat alone, staring out of the window: 'There was a sort of solemn isolation from an outward world,' wrote her father, whose prose style was usually quite down-to-earth. 'There was a room where in the high region of storm and wind she sat alone as it were, looking over the great plain, meditating from her window like one of her own Prophets looking towards Jerusalem. It was a scene fit for the most contemplative of human minds – it was *above* the earth. Its like will not form part of human thought again.' In his account to her mother, he recorded only one sentence spoken by his daughter on that occasion: '"If I had health," she said [to me] quietly, "I should be seeing what was going on in hospitals."'

Florence was on the mend.

CHAPTER SEVEN

'By pestilence perished before their time'

Much of the population of England in the 1850s lived in conditions reminiscent of the Scutari Barrack Hospital in its worst days, and in urban districts less than half of the children survived their fifth year. The urban poor in particular lived surrounded by filth on a scale probably unmatched anywhere in the world. The cities, their population swollen by unprecedented commercial success, teemed with horses and other animals and their dung heaps. In 1855 there were twenty-six cowsheds in the square mile of the City of London alone, and 266 cows. There were numerous urban workshops making use of every part of an animal's corpse, from the stomach to the skin. Until its repeal in 1851, a tax on windows had encouraged the construction of unventilated houses. The towns had few sewers; the well-off had cesspools but many of the poor threw their excrement into ditches or into the street. The viscous remains of human cadavers bulged out of the overloaded church graveyards into the streets and cellars nearby. Piped water supplies were often drawn from the river at the same point the sewage entered it, and the flow was so unreliable that until a decade ago every Englishman kept a water storage tank in his attic. As late as 1866, a cholera epidemic claimed 18,000 lives in one year.

In the year following Nightingale's breakdown, 1858, London was visited by a man-made calamity known as the Great Stink, when the River Thames proved quite incapable of removing the vast quantity of horrors poured into it. The smell was so bad near the river that railway travellers leaving London Bridge station were seized by attacks of vomiting. These conditions may have had a negative effect on the life expectancy of the general population, but they made a positive contribution to Nightingale's mental health and possibly to her survival. She could distract herself from her failure to get her full evidence published by grappling directly with civilian public health issues that were closely related to her experience at Scutari. Firstly, political interests were preventing further expenditure on improved sanitation in England saying that such improvements would not reduce the death rate, and secondly, the doctors were insisting that the

London hospitals should be located where they were convenient for *them*, not for the patients.

She was also working for reform of military hygiene, where she had influence at the War Office through Sidney Herbert. Her political influence in civilian life was not, on the surface of it, as strong; her ally William Farr did not even have the full backing of his civil service superiors on account of his edgy radical views. But informally, Nightingale was stronger than she appeared. When she picked herself up after her breakdown and took stock of her assets, she realised that she gained a new one. The government had suppressed scientific evidence, produced by its own civil servant Farr, of great importance to a public enquiry that it had authorised her to conduct, and which it had promised would be a full and open treatment of a matter of great public concern. The fact that the Cabinet had then suppressed that scientific evidence seemed to give credence to it, especially as that evidence pointed to the Cabinet being responsible for the disaster at Scutari rather than the army's High Command or its Medical Department. Florence Nightingale now had this suppressed evidence in her hands: the government's dirty little secret.

The buck did not stop with Sidney Herbert. It had been a coalition Cabinet, including all the leading political lights of the day including various Dukes and brothers of Earls and protégés of aristocrats, like Gladstone. All of them except Palmerston had muddled their portfolios so they were collectively responsible for the war's disasters. The post-war public mood was ugly, blaming the aristocracy and their cronies for mismanaging the war and then ending it too early when things seemed to be going Britain's way at last. If Florence Nightingale went public with her evidence, the result would be unpredictable and not good for the political elite. For this reason if no other, government officials and civil servants had to take her views on civilian public health seriously. She would soon show them that she was willing to drop the handkerchief at her window and bring the mob onto the streets.

She was up against the victorious medical opponents of Edwin Chadwick. When parliament had retired Chadwick and abolished his Board of Health just a few months before Nightingale went to war, there was an alternative and more politically acceptable national public health leader already waiting in the wings. This was the well-connected surgeon and pathologist John Simon, who had risen to prominence in the City of London and whom Chadwick had persuaded Lord Palmerston to drop from the Crimean Sanitary Commission. This decision was beneficial to Simon who was able to secure the post of national Chief Medical Officer while the commission was away at the war. Chadwick had proposed the absent Sutherland for the post, but as Chadwick's protégé he had no chance against Simon.

After Chadwick's fall, his allies saw their official careers blighted. Not surprisingly, the career doctors attached to the army in the Crimea attacked

Sutherland's Sanitary Commission, composed as it was of renegade doctors who had sided with Chadwick. Sutherland's report into Crimean War sanitation was not published until the war was over; immediately a pamphlet war broke out between Sutherland and Sir John Hall, the army's Principal Medical Officer, and his supporters. Hall alleged that Sutherland's Sanitary Commission had done nothing to reduce the death rate, while Nightingale trumpeted its achievements and Sutherland cautiously claimed partial success. The Crimean experience did not restore the prestige of the Chadwick school; by the time Sutherland's commission had completed its work, medical professionals under the leadership of John Simon had seized official control of public health and curbed what they perceived to be Chadwick's excesses.

John Simon, during his official leadership of the public health movement after 1855, tended to employ medical men on the way up the career ladder of that profession, on a temporary basis, rather than doctors and engineers committed to sanitation of the type favoured by Chadwick. He also spent a significant part of his public funds on medical research, and on his own admission regularly blinded his political masters with science to prevent them from controlling him. The low-tech Chadwick school did not prosper during the Simon era, fitting in as best they could in various underpaid niches of public life. Simon kept his private sector posts at St Thomas's Hospital, added to which he was one of the highest paid employees of the public sector at £2,000 a year.

Simon believed that disease could only be prevented when its causes had been discovered, and did not think that there was enough evidence to show how the 'miasma' that emanated from dirt caused epidemic disease (Simon, unlike Farr and Nightingale, was a miasmatist at the time). He argued that Government should devote more financial resources to medical research. Instead of *compelling* local authorities to clean up the cities, as Chadwick proposed, Simon wanted to *persuade* them to do so by using arguments based on superior knowledge obtained through research. It would be his highly paid job to acquire and deploy this superior knowledge. His philosophy fitted perfectly with the objectives of medical professionals, and was politically attractive because it did not involve compulsory measures. Chadwick had been criticised on the grounds that his centralising approach interfered with civil liberties, which at that time meant the powers of parish councils.

Nightingale and the Chadwick school claimed that Simon was pursuing knowledge and 'big science' for its own sake, and that like most medical men Simon was only interested in finding new ways of explaining what the patient had died from. 'What is needed now is not to know, but to do,' said Nightingale. In 1857, she replaced Chadwick as the spokesperson of the low-tech sanitarian movement. She had abandoned her loyalty to the doctors and had become, like Dr Sutherland and Dr Farr who had carefully recruited and groomed her for the task, a medical deserter. Nightingale knew that Chadwick's self-important and intolerant approach had alienated the whole nation and had stalled the compulsory public health movement that Chadwick himself had founded. The way to implement Chadwick's schemes was to remove all trace of the Chadwick approach. A soft, insidious, consensus building was needed, with no authoritarian discipline, no personality cult, and an emphasis on basic human values instead of money. It was not the price of soap that would convince Londoners to demand that soft, clean water be piped in from the Surrey hills, it was the fact that it would save their babies' lives.

Chadwick and Nightingale made an effective team, and it was Chadwick who suggested to her that she write a self-help guide for women explaining how they should care for a family's health at home. But she was in consternation when Chadwick wanted to help her to publicise the results of her Royal Commission on the health of the army by writing an article about army hygiene in an influential magazine. She wrote to Chadwick advising him to leave the medical profession's motives to the reader's own judgement: 'while stating the case and its remedies fully and openly to leave the inferences to us, the readers, as far as possible.' This was the woman who two years before had flung back in Sidney Herbert's teeth the advice he gave her to tone down her despatches in which she was attributing the darkest motives to Dr Hall, telling her that 'the public like to have something left to their own imaginations and are much pleased with their own sagacity when they have found out what was too obvious to be missed.' She had come a long way since the war. And Nightingale had one further piece of advice for Chadwick when he was drafting his article. She thought that it might be a good idea if the great sanitary leader, twenty years her senior, could for once address his readers 'as if you loved them'.

Her first public clash with Chadwick's rival John Simon came when Simon publicly supported the claim of Dr Edward Greenhow that improving sanitation could not reduce the high mortality from whooping cough, scarlet fever, and measles, three diseases that between them were killing half of all urban children before they reached the age of five. Simon had obtained the post of Lecturer in Public Health at St Thomas's Hospital for Greenhow, and published this claim in one of his official reports in 1858, approving Greenhow's finding that the horrific mortality from these fevers was, in Simon's words 'practically speaking, unavoidable.' Nightingale argued that premature death from these fevers could be almost entirely avoided by improvements to water supply, sewers, and ventilation of buildings, and she and Chadwick anonymously attacked Simon's official state-funded pronouncement in the press. Simon eventually retracted his statement in print, or rather pretended that he had never written it, but only twenty years later after he had resigned, by which time the issue was no longer in doubt.

Nightingale also attacked Simon's pronouncement by deploying her most famous coloured diagram, which she first published at this time in her *Contribution to the Sanitary History of the British Army*. This expensively produced coffee-table book was anonymous too, although it contained no confidential data, but no one could have any doubt about its authorship because of its subject matter and the fact that it made no reference to Nightingale at all, which would have been otherwise obligatory. The *Contribution* contained her first public announcement, in the accompanying text, that the wartime mortality statistics proved that sanitation would reduce premature mortality in Britain:

> Let us now ask, how was it that our noble army all but perished in the East? And we shall at the same time learn how it has happened that so many hundreds of millions of the human race have by pestilence perished before their time.

She included in this book her famous coloured diagram, now commonly known as the coxcomb; an improvement on one she had included in the Royal Commission report. It consists of two circles composed of wedges summarising the deaths from different causes in the first and second years of the war respectively. The Sanitary Commission began its work at the end of the first year, and the second year shows a marked reduction in deaths from epidemic disease showing that mortality can be controlled. The text points out that 'Similar diagrams might be produced for towns in their unimproved and improved state, and even for single buildings, inhabited by large numbers of persons.' She was using the diagram in a *prescriptive* way, to call for expenditure on sanitation in towns and buildings, rather than to simply show that most deaths in war are due to disease which is how modern commentators often interpret it. That would just be a *descriptive* message, but understanding the political context and the text accompanying it reveals that Nightingale was the first to use statistical graphics to support an argument for change. The diagram supported her argument that epidemic disease should be controlled by environmental improvements.

In the text accompanying her diagram, Nightingale criticised Simon and Greenhow and their description of scarlet fever mortality as unavoidable, accusing them of defective methodology. Nightingale also helped Chadwick to point out a logical flaw in Simon's argument in the pages of *The Builder*, a paper that gave space to the sanitarians. Simon had explained that the mortality from these fevers was unavoidable because 'Wherever human beings may cross one another's path, the susceptible person may contract the infection'. His mistake in logic was to assume that if it was inevitable that many people would *catch* the infection then it was also inevitable

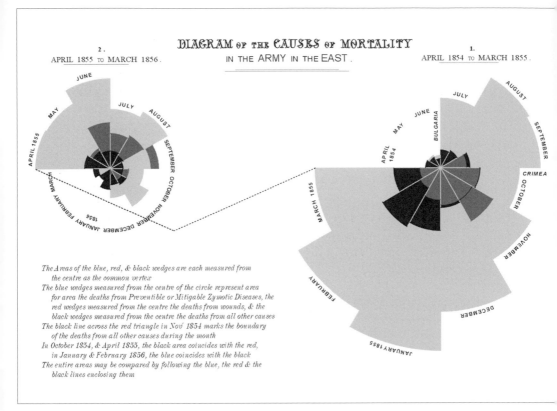

Nightingale's 'coxcomb' diagram illustrating the reduction in epidemic disease during the war.

that they would *die* from it. Simon partially contradicted himself on this point by saying that 'the fatality of these diseases is greatly and evidently proportionate to exterior conditions such as overcrowding and poor ventilation.' But in describing the mortality as unavoidable, Simon ignored this qualification. A clue to his apparent self-contradiction is his use of the word 'science': 'Liability to these infections is a more or less considerable risk which *science* hitherto cannot avert.' This sums up Simon's view of prevention, which was very different from Nightingale's. His definition of 'preventable' appeared to be that *science* could prevent it. He seemed to believe that overcrowding and poor ventilation were unalterable, but that science would eventually be able to compensate for them.

It was as if Simon dreamed that scientific discovery would be able to leapfrog over the political obstacles that caused so much trouble when public health officials had tried to improve the dwellings of the poor during the Chadwick era. It was a dream that was to lead to a lifetime's disappointment for John Simon, but it was not an irrational dream, as Louis Pasteur's achievements in France show. England passed temporary and unpopular laws compelling dog owners to muzzle their pets during the 1880s and 1890s, and succeeded in eliminating rabies in this way. But France did not do so, and used Pasteur's rabies vaccine as an alternative method of control. Simon would have preferred Pasteur's high-tech approach of attacking the disease itself rather than the conditions that produced it.

Simon's co-author Dr Greenhow wrote to *The Builder* warning against the exaggerated claims of the sanitarians: 'It is so very important that no false expectations of the benefits derivable from sanitary exertions should be raised in the public mind . . . There are, indeed, certain diseases which are preventable, but this does not apply to scarlet fever.' The letter concluded that the causes of mortality 'demand much careful investigation, and that, with certain exceptions, such investigation must precede any further progress in the art of preventing disease.' In this he was reiterating Simon's doctrine that 'Disease can only be prevented by those who have knowledge of its causes' and was effectively calling for a halt to sanitary expenditure and a diversion of funds to medical research. But scarlet fever was both preventable and mitigable; being a droplet infection it spreads more easily and takes a more severe course in poorly ventilated or overcrowded buildings, and ventilation was one of Nightingale's sanitary obsessions after the war. Greenhow failed to consider ventilation in his list of possible 'sanitarian exertions', and also failed to see that preventing a disease from being severe or fatal can be as beneficial as preventing it entirely.

At this time, the end of 1858, Nightingale's Royal Commission report was also failing to convince army doctors. They would not accept her conclusion that the disease originated in the hospitals, even less her recommendation that independent sanitary specialists should be attached to the army. The pamphlet war between military doctors and civilian sanitarians that had started with the publication of Sutherland's Sanitary Commission report in early 1857 had intensified. The army doctors claimed that the reduction in mortality in the middle of the war, which Nightingale's Royal Commission report claimed was due to improved sanitation, was due to other factors. Certainly, there was no direct evidence in her report to support her conclusion, because the government had suppressed it. At this point, with John Simon obstructing the civilian sanitarian movement and Sir John Hall opposing sanitary reform in the army, Nightingale decided it was time to give her opponents a glimpse of the cards she had in her hand. She paid for the printing of a large number of copies of her confidential report *Notes on Matters affecting the Health of the British Army*, which contained unpublished evidence on the public health disaster at Scutari. Farr's suppressed statistics were included, proving that poor building hygiene was the main cause of death. She sent it to 500 of the leading thinkers of the day including doctors, bishops, parliamentarians, and prominent business leaders. She marked it 'Confidential' and bound the recipients in a covering letter not to publicise it. When sending it to medical people, she included a second volume containing a 'Note on Contagion and Infection' in which she attacked Simon's pronouncement of 'inevitable mortality', which was so similar to the fatalistic and self-serving attitude of the doctors at the Scutari hospital. Nightingale wrote that this official pronouncement of the country's Chief Medical Officer was being used by the enemies of sanitation to block expenditure on sanitary schemes.

This very selective and limited leak of confidential information showed the recipients that the government had suppressed the findings of its supposedly public enquiry – she included the official letter from the Minister of War identifying it as a report commissioned by him. Any more trouble, they could conclude, and this would go to the press. Sir John Hall abruptly stopped his pamphleteering, army sanitary reform went ahead, and Dr Sutherland was paid a retainer by the new and independent Army Sanitary Committee for many years to come. John Simon remained in titular charge of state medicine but Chadwick and Nightingale shadowed him, successfully lobbying politicians to restrain Simon's excessively scientific and research-oriented approach.

Nightingale picked another high-profile quarrel with Simon practically straight away, this time over the location of a new hospital. The charity hospital of St Thomas's, where Simon had retained his post as senior surgeon, had to move when its site was required for a new railway station. Nightingale had established herself as an expert on hospital design through her articles in *The Builder,* and the authorities of the hospital sought her help in planning the replacement hospital. Nightingale and her sanitarians wanted the new hospital built in the London suburbs, as did some of the resident staff. She was convinced that a hospital in the suburbs surrounded by acres of parkland would be healthier than one in the centre of London, where in any case she maintained that there were already too many hospitals.

John Simon and other non-resident specialists wanted the charity hospital rebuilt on a central London site. They lobbied government officials for a town site and claimed that if the hospital moved to the suburbs then Simon and other 'practitioners of eminence' would not be able to provide emergency cover since their private patients required them to remain in central London close to the town houses of the rich. (Paying patients never went into hospital in those days, even for major surgery; it was far too dangerous.) A letter from Simon and others to *The Times* complained that if the hospital moved to the suburbs 'ultimate responsibility for the patients would fall on resident officers not engaged in private practice, with the result that the standard of skill would degenerate.' The hospital's resident doctors, after this amazing insult, mounted a counter-attack with their sanitary allies using statistics that showed that central London hospitals killed more of their patients than suburban ones.

Naturally, Farr and Nightingale were happy to provide statistical arguments for moving to the suburbs, using comparisons of the mortality of hospitals in London compared to those outside. They infuriated the medical profession by assuming in these comparisons that hospital hygiene was the only factor influencing patient mortality. This was an assumption based on the studies that Farr had seen in Paris into the mortality of armies in the Mediterranean, and on the lesson of Scutari. The darker, more sinister belief lurking in the shadows was the idea that the main beneficiaries of the central London hospitals were the rich patients of society surgeons and physicians like John Simon who were practising their skills on the sick poor in hospital so as to better treat the rich in their safe townhouses. This argument was never far from the surface of Nightingale's later popular writings.

When she threw in her lot with St Thomas's, Nightingale seems to have compromised Sidney Herbert's plan to use the Nightingale Fund to train female hospital nurses. The resident staff at St Thomas's agreed to let her design the new hospital, provided that she allowed the Fund's student nurses to work while studying. When, during the war, Nightingale had accepted responsibility for the Fund which was to bear her name, the object had been to provide an institute for training hospital nurses independently. When she returned from the war, she postponed a decision on how to use the money, and after the Royal Commission was over and she had recovered from her collapse she suddenly wanted nothing more to do with it because hospital nursing was no longer her highest priority.

Herbert had launched the Nightingale Fund by reading aloud at a public meeting a letter from a soldier describing how he and his comrades in the Scutari hospital kissed Nightingale's shadow as she passed. With this beginning, it would not be surprising if the new Florence Nightingale felt oppressed by the responsibility she had accepted for the Fund. Press, public, and politicians bombarded her with demands that she dedicate the rest of her life to carrying out the original nursing objectives of the Fund in a teaching hospital and under the supervision of the medical profession. It must have seemed to her as if she was being pressured to dedicate her life to repeating the errors of Scutari. Not surprisingly, she tried to resign from her position with the Fund, but Herbert would not allow it. It may have been partly in desperation, to ensure that wild horses could not drag her back to work in a hospital, that she took to her bed. By 1859, she was claiming that her health prevented her from supervising the use of the Fund, although at the time she was working flat out to oppose John Simon's pronouncements. When Herbert began to organise a nurse training school in Kings College Hospital, it spurred Nightingale into action at

St Thomas's. She effectively traded the Fund for the right to design the new hospital, in accordance with her new building hygiene priorities. For Nightingale, the hospital was to be a temporary expedient – necessary for the 150 years or so that it would take to upgrade ordinary people's homes and make them safer for the care of the sick than any hospital could be. It would be a safe version of the Scutari Barrack Hospital – a general hospital in the clean London suburbs, 'remote from the battlefield' to which patients would be carried from the city by Brunel's new railways which were the perfect replacement for the ghastly hospital transport ships of the Black Sea.

The hospital did not move to the suburbs, because John Simon defeated Nightingale and the resident staff and managed to get it built on the banks of the Thames opposite the Houses of Parliament where it was convenient for both his private practice and his political career. The Nightingale Fund set up its nurse training school there but Nightingale ignored its activities, claiming to be incapacitated by illness. She did succeed in designing the new buildings, using her favourite scheme of many separate 'pavilions' to improve ventilation. Her buildings still stand, despite the frequent appearance of projects for their replacement. Whatever the sanitary advantages, her pavilion plan proved useful in limiting bomb damage during the Second World War, only a few of the pavilions being badly damaged. The bombs missed Florence Nightingale's archives which were stored in the hospital, but destroyed those of John Simon. Simon would be better known to posterity if he had agreed to the hospital site on forty acres of parkland in Lewisham that Nightingale had favoured.

Nightingale and Chadwick dogged Simon's footsteps for years, using all their efforts to keep the sanitarian movement out of his hands and to combat his theories and doctrines. Eventually, in 1871, they persuaded the Cabinet to relieve Simon of most of his powers and to put official leadership of public health back into the hands of the practical sanitarians. In their letter to the Cabinet Minister, which prompted this decision, Chadwick and Nightingale wrote 'men with theories have absolutely no place in sanitary administration.'

In 1887, after his retirement, John Simon reprinted the 1858 paper that annoyed Nightingale so much and surreptitiously retracted his claim that mortality was unavoidable. Simon kept the date of June 1858 in this reprint, and his editor claimed that 'the revision of the proof sheets by Mr Simon himself has been for the purpose of giving clearer expression to his original meaning and not for the purpose of altering his opinions which were founded upon the existing state of knowledge at the time.' Despite this claim, Simon radically altered the text. For example, he deleted some passages in which he had cast doubt on Dr John Snow's then recent discovery that cholera spread through drinking water. At the time, he had refused to accept Snow's simple 'unscientific' proof based on observation of the results of different water supplies to different houses. 'We must wait for scientific insight,' Simon had characteristically told his employers in the City of London. In the 1887 reprint, Simon also altered his original 1858 statement that the deaths from measles, whooping cough, and scarlet fever are 'practically speaking, unavoidable', to read 'in some degree, unavoidable'. Nightingale would have found it hard to quarrel with that.

How much did the practical sanitarians achieve? Did Nightingale and her sanitarian followers succeed in putting the lessons of Scutari to good use? A debate has been continuing for decades about what caused the steep increase in life expectancy in Britain after the Crimean War – from thirty-nine years in the late 1850s to fifty-five when Nightingale died in 1910. This is the steepest rise in modern history, and in the 1970s Thomas McKeown published a groundbreaking study that showed that advances in medical treatment made no contribution to the decline in mortality in those years. His evidence showed that the mortality from epidemics such as whooping cough, measles, and scarlet fever, which John Simon had said was unavoidable, fell dramatically during that period before any medical treatment or vaccine for these diseases was available. This part of his conclusion is still widely accepted, but his demonstration that the increase in life expectancy must have been due primarily to rising living standards enabling better nutrition is not. He chose nutrition not on any direct evidence but by eliminating other possible causes.

McKeown eliminated the hypothesis that microbes declined in virulence by saying that six different microbes would not all choose the same moment to mutate into weaker strains. He eliminated the hypothesis that natural selection might have created human immunity by pointing out that there had been no previous surge in mortality signalling that the less immune individuals were being eliminated from the gene pool. The final possibility was that sanitary exertions had reduced the mortality from the common fevers. He gave some of the credit to sanitation, but argued that the sanitarians could not have reduced mortality from droplet infections like scarlet fever because such diseases are not spread by water supply or sewage. McKeown omitted to note that the sanitarians (particularly Nightingale) included the improvement of ventilation among their priorities; McKeown was guilty of the same error that Dr Greenhow had made in 1858. Taking this into account, it is likely that improved sanitation counted for as much as improved nutrition in the dramatic reduction in mortality after the Crimean War. McKeown, a medical academic, wanted to apply his findings to the problem of premature mortality in underdeveloped countries. The British experience between 1850 and 1900 may be still relevant in that context, but it is clear that increasing longevity in Britain today owes much more to medical therapy and pharmacology.

Recently, anthropologists, archaeologists, and others have produced independent evidence of the impact of sanitation and nutrition on mortality. Archaeology has revealed that when humans began to give up their hunter-gatherer lifestyle after the spread of agriculture about 10,000 years ago, the health of our species went into rapid decline and life expectancy decreased. This was due to a more monotonous diet and the fact that the sedentary farmers lived surrounded by effluent and newly domesticated animals which were reservoirs of disease. The human frame was not designed for dense ant-like colonies or a limited diet, and skeletons of sedentary dwellers show the ravages of disease and poor nutrition. Paradoxically, though, the human population increased rapidly because giving up the mobile hunter-gatherer existence in favour of settlement allowed a woman to produce children more frequently. As population densities increased, health continued to decline until a tipping-point was reached when the industrial revolution caused a migration of the rural population to the cities of Victorian Britain, and mortality skyrocketed. What the sanitarians did, instead of restoring the hunter-gatherers' mobility, was to make the *effluent* mobile and to ban farm animals and graveyards from the towns.

Was this pure luck? Did the sanitarians 'do the right thing for the wrong reasons' while scientists like Simon and Greenhow unfairly had to struggle along the hard road of true enlightenment towards technological development? Not exactly; the sanitarians were not entirely motivated by superstitious ideas that smell equals disease. Nightingale shows in her *Contribution* that history already provided evidence that supported her movement: 'Were we able to follow the history of the town as it increased in size, and sanitary precautions were neglected, we should find the wedges of our diagram getting larger and larger, until, in the course of years, the town might become almost uninhabitable, as has been the case with many ancient cities.'

Another, more individual contribution that Nightingale made to reducing premature mortality was in keeping the poor out of hospital. By the time she had lost her battle over the location of the new St Thomas's, Nightingale had written a best-selling book which flew over the head of the nation's Chief Medical Officer and into the minds of the only people who could keep the population away from doctors and their hospitals entirely: the housewives and domestic servants of England.

Published in 1860, *Notes on Nursing* sold 15,000 copies in its first two months, and has never been out of print in the 140 years since. Many of its early readers must have been baffled to discover that their two shillings had bought them something other than what the title and the author's reputation seemed to promise. Many of them must have been hoping for advice on what to expect from a career in hospital nursing, the profession that Nightingale had made so fashionable. Instead they got a radical anti-nursing, anti-medical, anti-hospital propaganda pamphlet. Lytton Strachey, in *Eminent Victorians,* noted the anti-nursing bias of Nightingale's best-seller, calling it a 'compendium of the besetting sins of the sisterhood, drawn up with the detailed acrimony, the vindictive relish, of a Swift.' Many a reader must have been bewildered by the first sentence of the book's preface, and turned back to the cover to see whether this was the book that she had intended to buy: 'The following notes are by no means intended as a rule of thought by which nurses can teach themselves to nurse, still less as a manual to teach nurses to nurse.'

What on earth is this book then? The answer, 'hints for thought to women who have charge of the health of others' is perplexing. What is such a woman if she is not a nurse? The answer was: she is *Everywoman.*

Within the first dozen pages, the reader learns that professional hospital nurses have been trained to obstruct God's reparative processes and that children's hospitals increase child mortality. The reader – Everywoman – finds herself ridiculed for her belief that 'nature intended mothers to be accompanied by doctors'. Later, she learns that doctors cannot agree which is their ethical duty: to alleviate the suffering of a patient who has an interesting medical condition, or to let the suffering continue so that they can observe it. Unfortunately, the manuscript drafts of this first edition have disappeared, otherwise we would be able to see why the non-confrontational Dr Sutherland was so alarmed by the anti-medical bias of the opening pages that he persuaded Nightingale to tone them down. What we see now is the censored version.

The book was targeted at women in domestic service who might have to care for the sick in their homes. From the 1851 census, Nightingale had discovered that nearly two thirds of the nurses in Britain were working in domestic service in private houses. Half of these nurses were nineteen years old or younger. This explains the simplistic language of the book, which may jar to the modern reader. The book also loses much of its effect today because it was written in an era where fatal sickness was a familiar resident in every household. Twenty-three in every 1000 of the population were dying every year, mostly from the fevers and infections that cause us no more than minor inconvenience, now that the annual death rate is more like nine in 1000. Nightingale wanted her book to keep people out of hospital and to downgrade the role of physicians in the eyes of ordinary people. Doctors, she wrote, do not cure. The human body cures itself, doctors may be called on to perform a kind of 'surgery of functions' analogous to a surgeon's task of removing a bullet from a wound so that the body's reparative processes can act. She never properly explains this 'surgery of functions', and most of the anecdotes about physicians in the book do not reflect to their credit. She has more praise for surgeons – a typical anecdote shows a surgeon opening the windows and a physician then closing them to the detriment of the patients – something that Nightingale claimed actually happened at Scutari.

She dismissed with a few short and equivocal remarks the traditional profession of nursing with which her readers identified her – the application of poultices, administration of medicines, care of bedsores, prevention of bleeding etc. She notes its value, but then spoils this tribute by saying that few patients die for lack of it. True nursing, she writes, should from now on be defined as 'the proper use of fresh air, light, warmth, cleanliness, quiet, and the proper selection and administration of diet – all at the least expense of vital power to the patient.'

Her book did not accuse the doctors of fraud and conspiracy, but blamed her readers for delegating too much authority to them. She did not attach herself to any of the strong anti-medical movements of the day. She was in favour of the compulsory smallpox vaccination, for example, whereas the most virulently anti-medical campaigners of the time were anti-vaccinationists who accused the medical profession of the most awful crimes under cover of the compulsory programme that had existed (in theory) since the 1820s. But the book shows signs that Nightingale may have believed in a medical conspiracy even if she preferred not to base her campaign on it. She notes that if her readers follow her advice they will reduce the work of doctors, and adds rather too jauntily that no doctor could possibly object to this. And she claims that some doctors would not interfere if they thought that a patient was being accidentally poisoned by a copper kettle, for fear of losing a mine of information. The book helped to promote the grass-roots change in public perception of health care that is now widely credited with helping to reduce premature mortality.

Although Nightingale's anti-medical bias in the years immediately after the Crimean War was influenced by Farr's attitudes, she was not his mouthpiece. She did not, to put it mildly, share Farr's admiration for John Simon, but she did benefit enormously from Farr's insights as a qualified physician. She later destroyed the written evidence of her education by Farr. Not knowing this, commentators have often treated Nightingale's medical and sanitary ideas as shallow because they do not believe she did enough research to have a proper theoretical foundation. For instance, Lytton Strachey in *Eminent Victorians* says that if Nightingale's experience had been treating yellow fever in Panama instead of cholera *(sic)* at Scutari she would have spent the rest of her life maintaining that the only way to deal with disease was by destroying mosquitoes. A little practical knowledge, he implies, was for her a dangerous thing. Strachey's error was in supposing that Nightingale learned anything at all about sanitation at Scutari. She learned her lesson afterwards, analysing highly complex data in a room in the Burlington Hotel in Mayfair, under the tutorship of one of the best medical scholars in the world. There, she drained the cup of knowledge to its bitterest dregs.

Understanding the change in her motivation and the development of her knowledge after the war helps enormously to extract meaning from her writings. Much of her output before her post-war breakthrough, or breakdown, can be discounted. She was naïve, intelligent, compassionate, and competitive, and she tended to echo the ideas of whoever was the most impressive man she had met so far. Afterwards, she became her own man, wiser, self-effacing, an unbiased judge of character and a skilled politician. We should read more carefully exactly what she said about public health after the war, because it was informed by experience few others would ever have. It makes it very hard to give the later Nightingale the necessary attention if one confuses her with the rather shrill and vehement character of her wartime years.

Nightingale's refusal to rely exclusively on 'germ theory' in public health has been cited as evidence that she was not scientific, even though her teacher William Farr was ahead of the field in anticipating germ theory. Medical historians have, for example, directly criticised her for her 'overconfident' diagnoses that the deaths of Sidney Herbert and Lord Raglan were related to their emotional problems. She claimed that Herbert died of regret at not having succeeded in reorganising the War Office of which he was the chief. And according to her, Raglan had turned his face to the wall in the Crimea and died of regret at his failure as Commander-in-Chief, his condition being aggravated by his maintenance of a calm outward appearance. It is remarkable that in Raglan's case she diagnosed repressed guilt, a diagnosis which must have seemed far-fetched at the time but which is a plausible explanation of her own behaviour.

Nightingale was largely bedridden for several years after 1861, reportedly suffering severe joint pains, palpitations, and other physical symptoms. Some have attributed her illness to psychosomatic causes; others have claimed that she faked her symptoms to manipulate people or to ensure seclusion so that she could work harder. To counter both of these suggestions, Dr David Young advanced a new diagnosis in a 1995 article in the British Medical Journal. Young was the first to propose an organic illness as the cause of Nightingale's invalidism. He showed that her varied and intermittent physical symptoms resembled a chronic form of brucellosis infection.

Young was an admirer of Nightingale, and he made it clear that to defend her reputation he only needed to show that neurosis or faking are not the only possible explanations for her physical symptoms. If he succeeded in showing that there was an organic illness that could have caused her sporadic and varied symptoms, it wouldn't prove that she had it, and it wouldn't disprove the earlier theories, but it would make it clear that they were pure speculation. Young's analysis was convincing thanks to Nightingale's well-documented attack of fever in the Crimea, which he showed to be very much like an attack of brucellosis. This infectious disease was common in the Mediterranean basin at that time and was transmitted in goat's milk, which civilians in the Crimea could afford as a substitute for cow's milk. But an attack of brucellosis only rarely leads to an extended period of chronic symptoms, so it is still only a speculative diagnosis of her later symptoms; that was all Young needed to rebut an allegation that there was no possible cause of her symptoms. And, most importantly, Young does not make any comment on the origin of her so-called depression.

This so-called depression was much more continuous and long-lasting than her other symptoms. According to Young, she suffered a continuous 25 year period of what he called 'depression, with feelings of worthlessness and failure'. Although depression is listed in the textbooks as a possible symptom of brucellosis, the same textbooks make it clear that most brucellosis patients do not have depression. So although, as Young said, depression was 'consistent' with brucellosis, absence of depression would be even more consistent with brucellosis. Even if present, depression may be caused by something else, and so the medical authorities cited in Young's paper warn against assuming that depression in a brucellosis sufferer is caused by that infection. This, and the fact that her feelings of worthlessness went on for a decade after physical symptoms had stopped, must be why Young deliberately avoided saying that her mental state was due to brucellosis. His guarded conclusion was that it was possible that 'chronic brucellosis condemned Florence to a lifetime of confinement and pain', conspicuously excluding her mental state from the symptoms explained.

Apart from the fact that Young did not attribute her 'feelings of worthlessness and failure' to brucellosis, it is unlikely that he thought they were a part of a wider form of depression. An 'inappropriate' feeling of worthlessness and failure is only one symptom from the list of nine officially cited by the American Psychiatric Association of which at least five are needed to justify a diagnosis of major depression. Young did not cite any other symptoms of depression, although he did mention cold and heartless personal relationships and a cruel, tyrannical and reproachful attitude. Regardless of whether his source (Woodham-Smith) exaggerated these traits, they are not symptoms either of depression or of brucellosis. At the time Young wrote his paper, it was not known that Nightingale had recognised her mistake over the cause of high mortality in her hospital. Young, like all other historians at the time, thought that she was a national heroine for having dramatically reduced the death rate. If Young had known about her shocking discovery he might not have concluded that her feelings of failure were inappropriate enough to constitute an isolated depressive symptom.

Biographical studies have shown that before the war Nightingale had a nearly complete set of symptoms of depression. So it seems that if she ever had depression, the war cured it. This would not be surprising given the torture she was released from by achieving her independence and a mission in life.

A diagnosis of depression is also incompatible with the productivity that Nightingale displayed during the post-war years. Even if one assumes, like some of her detractors, that her work was of little value, the sheer weight of paper input and output makes it an unbelievable feat from someone suffering from continuous depression. This productivity was one motivation for the essays by Mackowiak and others in 2005 and 2007, diagnosing her as suffering from bipolar disorder, also known as manic depression. However, Mackowiak's evidence for depression and mania is from before the war, including the only evidence presented that Nightingale was subject to the irrational elation characteristic of the manic stage, which was her 1853 statement 'I am now in the heyday of my power'. He cannot be correct in construing this statement as irrational because at the time she was chief executive of a hospital and one of the most powerful independent women in Britain.

Another indicator of Nightingale's freedom from depression is that sufferers have a diminished ability to concentrate and have disturbed cognitive processes. They can't think straight. Nightingale's reasoning ability, demonstrated by her detection of the logical flaws in John Simon's argument against practical sanitary measures, show that her cognitive processes were of high order.

Her dependence on logical reasoning and empirical methods was a consequence of Unitarian influence. Many of her public health pronouncements reflect the Unitarian emphasis on 'deeds not creeds'. Her comment disparaging John Simon's call for more research is a good example that has already been quoted: 'What is needed now is not to know, but to do'. Her strong antipathy to medical dogma, which drove her to reject unproven theory even when she didn't have a better replacement, reflects a Unitarian position. John Simon's theories, like the Church of England's creed, acted as a loyalty test that those seeking public funding or patronage had to pass, and in doing so had to recognise the superior insight and authority of the hierarchy. Unitarians were more worried about the Church of England's abuse of power and its use of the creed as a loyalty

test for teachers and other public servants than about the truth *per se* of
its doctrine of the Trinity. Nightingale's brand of Unitarianism claimed
that ordinary logic and observation were enough to reveal that benevolent
forces are at work throughout the universe. From this she could infer that
the Supreme Being is infinitely wise and benevolent, and what wiser and
more benevolent way to create man than to give him the means to create
himself? It is not surprising to learn that the young Charles Darwin was
taught by Unitarians. In his *Origin of Species*, published one month before
Notes on Nursing in 1859, Darwin showed by logic and observation how
all living species can create themselves.

She found another unusual outlet for her spirituality. By 1858, her
mystical devotion to the army's dead had already produced some strange
works of art – her famous statistical diagrams. She had persuaded Herbert
to include in the commission's report an annex containing coloured
diagrams of the mortality of the army, so that she could publish it as a
separate book, which would have the authority of Government by virtue
of the statement 'Reprinted from the Report of the Royal Commission'
on the title page. She thought that this colourful book would have more
impact on the military authorities than hundreds of pages of text, and she
had 2,000 copies printed on higher-quality paper and with more ornate
type than that used in the official report.

One of the more unusual diagrams in this book is a visual poem
illustrating the Royal Commission's main conclusion that the mortality
of the army in peacetime was too high. She and William Farr showed
that the mortality of soldiers in barracks at home in Britain was twice
as high as in the civilian districts which surrounded them, despite the
fact that army recruits were volunteers who were selected for their good
state of health. The statistics showed that if the army mortality could
be brought down to civilian levels, 1,200 soldiers' lives could be saved
every year. As she put it, 1,200 soldiers were being killed by bad barrack
sanitation every year just as if the army were taking 1,200 fit young
recruits out onto Salisbury Plain every year and shooting them. This
was the conclusion that the Royal Commission under Sidney Herbert
wanted to emphasise, to focus on continuing evils and opportunities
for improvement rather than investigating too closely the cause of past
'delinquencies' in the Crimea.

In her 1857 book of statistical diagrams, Nightingale's visual poem
to peacetime barracks mortality consists of four rhyming couplets of
horizontal bars, the first bar of each couplet being black and the second,
longer, being red. Each pair of bars represents the death rate of English
males in one of the four five-year age brackets between twenty and forty
years. The black bar represents civilians and the second (nearly twice as
long) represents soldiers in peacetime, in their barracks in England. At the

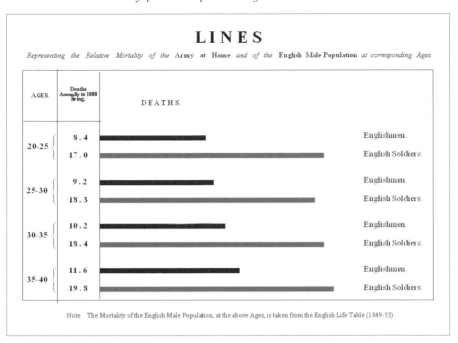

LINES

Representing the Relative Mortality of the Army *at* Home *and of the* English Male Population *at corresponding Ages*

AGES.	Deaths Annually to 1000 living.	DEATHS.	
20-25	8.4		Englishmen.
	17.0		English Soldiers.
25-30	9.2		Englishmen.
	18.3		English Soldiers.
30-35	10.2		Englishmen.
	18.4		English Soldiers.
35-40	11.6		Englishmen.
	19.8		English Soldiers.

Note   The Mortality of the English Male Population, at the above Ages, is taken from the English Life Table (1849-53)

'Our soldiers enlist to die in the barracks'. Peacetime mortality was mostly due to respiratory illness aggravated by poor ventilation.

end of each black bar is one word: *Englishmen*; at the end of each red bar, two words: *English Soldiers*. The thin rectangular coloured bars are reminiscent of the engraved maps of famous battlefields, where red British rectangles face off against darker colours to illustrate the positions of the forces at various stages of the battle. The red bar also brings to mind the famous Thin Red Line of Balaclava, where a two-deep line of red-jacketed British riflemen had turned back a horde of grey-clad Russian heavy cavalry bearing down on them, and thus saved the port and its vulnerable hospitals and stores behind them. On Nightingale's chart and under her command the Thin Red Line rose again, this time from the grave, to pour its deadly fire into the Army High Command.

Arthur Clough must have helped her to produce these diagrams, and it is intriguing to think that this one in particular may be a lost poem by the author of *Say not the struggle nought availeth*. The chart is headed *Lines* in ornate script, followed by the businesslike 'Representing the Relative Mortality of the Army at Home and of the English Male Population at Corresponding Ages'. The word 'Lines' recalls the title commonly used in Victorian poems, as in *Lines on the Death of Bismarck*. There is no logical reason for repeating the pictorial message four times, except for rhythmic and poetic effect. The rhythmic effect is provided by the words at the end of each bar, whose cadence recalls the harsh rattle of a kettledrum, beating alone in a soldier's funeral procession: 'English men, English soldiers, English men, English soldiers, English men . . .'

Nightingale spent large sums from the family fortune in privately printing deluxe editions of this type of material, commemorating the dead and recording the signs by which God was revealing to her the laws of sanitary progress. It has already been shown that one of the books, her 1859 *Contribution to the Sanitary History of the British Army*, first revealed her most famous 'coxcomb' diagram to the public and declared war on John Simon's doctrine that the current high mortality from epidemic disease was unavoidable. Another purpose of the book was to establish Nightingale as *the* authority on Crimean mortality, and point out the flaws in every other official and unofficial source. She had made herself the guardian of the mortality statistics.

In her obsessive exhibition of these statistical relics in graphical form, Nightingale had become Nemesis, or at least a priestess of the cult of that ancient goddess. Nemesis, in Greek mythology, was the daughter of Night and the grandchild of Chaos. She was the goddess of vengeance, persecutor of those who insulted the relics and the memory of the dead. She was also charged with punishing those mortals who are too proud, visiting them with losses and sufferings so that they may become humble. Few mortals can have been more severely punished by the gods for excessive pride than was Florence Nightingale. Now she was to become an avenger in her turn. She was the only one of her family to be born and to die with the name Nightingale. Her father's name was Shore; he had changed it when he inherited the Nightingale fortune. His family thereafter called him Night. Florence, like Nemesis, was the daughter of Night, who in mythology rode in a chariot drawn by owls and bats. An owl visited and spoke to Nightingale during the war, it will be remembered, when she was at her most complacent, watching the sun set gloriously over the masts of the British fleet on the evening before the arrival of the Sanitary Commission at her hospital. She thought at the time that her talkative nocturnal visitor was the ghost of an owl that she had once kept as a pet.

But Nightingale was to go further than merely guarding the relics. After the suppression of her confidential report in 1857, she received extensive support from the War Office for her scheme to eliminate the excess peacetime mortality in the barracks. The government, at Nightingale's request, appointed Herbert chair of the four sub-commissions that were formed in the wake of the Royal Commission into the Health of the Army. One of these was to make visits of inspection to all the army barracks in the land and authorise the immediate expenditure of money on sanitary improvements where needed. Sidney Herbert himself undertook these barrack inspections in the face of great hostility from the army officers. Herbert's health was failing fast – he was suffering from acute nephritis, quite possibly a delayed consequence of a violent scarlet fever epidemic in the crowded and unsanitary dormitories at Harrow, the exclusive boarding school that he had attended.

It is hard to imagine a less congenial task for one of the richest men in England than that of barrack sanitary inspector, even if he had been in good health. But as Nightingale said, she had a hold over Sidney Herbert. She set him the task of eliminating the excess mortality in the barracks, which she and Farr had calculated at 1,200 soldiers per year. If this result could be achieved then the lesson of Scutari would have been put to use, proving that 'your mistakes are part of God's plan'. The advantage of soldiers from the statistical point of view was that they were as near as possible interchangeable. In Nightingale's scheme, by reducing barracks mortality to civilian levels she and Sidney Herbert could each year bring 1,200 common soldiers back from the dead.

In mid-1859, after Herbert had spent two years trudging around dingy barracks inspecting drains under the hostile glare of the army dinosaurs, Palmerston appointed him Minister of War. Sidney Herbert was not the obvious choice; he was still blamed by many for the errors of the first winter in the Crimea, which Palmerston and had corrected after Herbert left office. But Palmerston in 1859 needed to put together a coalition and he needed members of other parties including Gladstone. Sidney Herbert was a protégé of Gladstone, who must have thought that his ailing friend deserved something better than the drudgery that Nightingale was imposing on him.

Nightingale did not mean to let Herbert off the hook. Now that he was War Minister she wanted him to carry out a complete reorganisation of the War Office. Without this, any army health reforms that Nightingale and Herbert had implemented would not become permanent. The War Office seems to have been lacking an organisation chart – everybody in it gave their opinion on every question and nobody seemed to have authority or accountability for any decision. The nearest thing in modern life would perhaps be the incompetent Town Hall of a scandal-prone London borough, as portrayed in the most lurid press accounts. The reorganisation of the War Office was obviously not a task for which Herbert was suited; he had no skill in administration or in outwitting his obstructive civil servants, who were often in thrall to rival politicians. When Herbert's illness was diagnosed as fatal in early 1861, he tried to persuade Nightingale to agree that he should resign as Minister of War. She talked him out of it. For the next six months he argued with his War Office subordinates over the plans for reorganisation. In June he collapsed and she accepted that he would resign, although she claimed that after two years' rest he would be able to get back to work.

At the beginning of August 1861, Sidney Herbert died, aged fifty-one, at his magnificent country estate of Wilton. It was four years to the day since his agreement with Nightingale that he would dedicate himself to saving soldiers' lives. At 1,200 per year, that would be 4,800 lives – the same as the number of soldiers who died in Nightingale's hospital at Scutari. But they had not yet started to pay off the debts of Balaclava General, the hospital ships, and the rest of the 16,000 unnecessary deaths. According to Nightingale, Herbert's dying words were: 'Poor Florence; our joint work unfinished.'

Her harsh treatment of Herbert continued after his death, when his distraught widow wanted to publish an article praising his achievements. Liz Herbert asked Gladstone, who had been Herbert's political mentor and was now Chancellor of the Exchequer, to persuade Nightingale to help with this article. Gladstone sent Nightingale a draft and asked for what he quaintly called 'numbers and other statistics' to support its claims. Gladstone told Nightingale that Liz Herbert believed that her husband would rather be remembered for having saved soldiers lives than for anything else. Nightingale did not have much sympathy for this desire to achieve immortality through personal fame. Herbert, she once said, 'Never said "I did this"' about something he had achieved. It was the trait she admired most in him and, after the war, went out of her way to emulate.

She wrote to Gladstone that Herbert would much rather the newspapers published Herbert's (i.e. her) plan for War Office reorganisation so that it would have some chance of succeeding, instead of the proposed eulogy. As to the successes claimed in Liz's article, such as the Royal Sanitary Commission, Nightingale alleged that most of them were due to another man. Of all people, Nightingale gave the credit to the previous Minister of War, Lord Panmure. This was a cruel cut at Gladstone, who was held in contempt by Lord Panmure for helping to persuade Lord Aberdeen to start the war and then wanting to sue for an early and humiliating peace before even having taken Sebastopol. It also sounds hypocritical given that Nightingale, before her conversion, could never mention Lord Panmure's name without going into paroxysms of spite because of his supposed cowardly treatment of McNeill and Tulloch and his obstruction of her Royal Commission.

She heaped praise on Lord Panmure with a trowel when rebuffing Gladstone's request for help with Liz Herbert's proposed eulogy of her husband. She told Gladstone that Herbert's lifetime of dedication to the British soldier, as described by Liz, had an unexplained two-year gap in it from March 1855 (when Herbert left the government) to February 1857, during which time she implied that Herbert had gone fishing and ignored her own efforts towards army reform. She wrote her own short analysis of Herbert's later achievements as an alternative to the widow's eulogy. In this piece, she gratuitously reminds readers that Herbert had been blamed for the disasters in the Crimea and then describes at length Lord Panmure's role in identifying and remedying them. Panmure had organised the Royal Commission that Herbert had chaired, and in case anyone should say that superiors should not get all the credit she pointed out that Herbert in turn had his own subordinates to do the real work.

She sent this masterpiece to Gladstone saying that she had not been able to think of a way to leave out mention of his enemy Lord Panmure without giving Panmure an opportunity to complain. She would be glad if Gladstone could help her to find a way to eliminate the former War Minister from her article, because 'the name of Panmure is an abomination in my ears'. This was well crafted irony. Gladstone must have known that she had criticised his enemy Panmure in the past, but even in her most spiteful period she would never have used biblical language of the type often affected by Gladstone himself. She offered to brief Chancellor of the Exchequer Gladstone on three important areas where government action would be much appreciated by his late protégé Sidney Herbert, and also hinted that Gladstone himself as a senior Minister at the time was even more responsible than Herbert for the loss of the army in the Crimea. Gladstone wrote back thanking her for her summary of Herbert's career and informing her that the family had decided not to publish a eulogy for the moment. As for the briefing she offered, he did not think he would be able to master the details of such an intricate subject. He withdrew from Nightingale's orbit and returned to his primary tasks of trimming the national budget and proving to his own satisfaction that Homer was a Christian. Nightingale later assessed Gladstone as 'the most unsanitary brute that ever was.'

In public, Nightingale's adulation of her dear departed master Sidney Herbert remained unbounded, but it appears that she wanted to stop Liz Herbert's eulogy so that she alone could exploit Sidney Herbert's memory in pursuit of her own objective of reforming the War Office. She had urged Herbert to continue working even when he was dying. She believed that she was dying herself, and given a probable earlier attack of brucellosis it seems likely that her painful symptoms were genuine, but she worked on obsessively in the face of repeated warnings and advice to rest from doctors including Sutherland, who had become her amanuensis as well as personal physician. She could not yet see any concrete results from her efforts to achieve a sanitary revolution in the face of John Simon's opposition, and she was panic-stricken at the magnitude of the task she felt compelled to undertake as the result of the government's failure to publish her vindication of the practical sanitarians. With the spectre of Scutari staring at her from the corner of her room – perhaps one of those young corpses she had gazed upon so calmly in the dead-house – she had no alternative course open to her except to succeed in her work at whatever cost. Others might have done the same in the circumstances.

Harder to explain than her relationship with Herbert was the one she had with Dr Sutherland, who had led the Crimean Sanitary Commission and with whom she spent more time than anyone else after the war. Sometimes she treated him as if he was her arch-enemy even though he was practically her slave for the rest of his life. When they were not on speaking terms he used to attend her anyway and she would pass notes to him across the room or under the door, sometimes conducting entire conversations this way. When he once told her that he could not come because he had some work to do on his garden she nearly expired with stupefied rage. But theirs was a productive symbiosis. She found him lucrative employment with the Army Sanitary Committee, which was her fiefdom entirely independent of the military authorities, until long after his normal retirement age. She moved to Hampstead for a while to be near to him, and when she moved to South Street in Mayfair she conceived the idea that he should come to live next door. It seems that she was on very good terms with his wife, but even so that idea did not appeal. She became very dependent on him, and often accepted his sensible advice to water down some of her more confrontational writings for publication. But she was very critical of him, and not only in private; once she wrote rebuking a correspondent who had 'flattered' Sutherland by telling him that he looked ill: 'Clough said Sutherland was a selfish brute and might have added "with a devil of a temper". Sutherland's mania is to be considered an invalid. He does nothing. The truth would be to tell him "you are killing Florence by letting her do everything that you don't like to do".'

Did she have something against Sutherland? A conjectural explanation is that when he was in the Crimea he 'saved the army' as she put it, by his improvements in sanitation, but did not tell her what had been wrong, never advised her that her hospital had been a 'pest-house' as she later described it. Much less confrontational than McNeill, he allowed Nightingale to go on broadcasting McNeill's theory that the men had been already dying when they arrived. And when his report appeared it did not, unlike McNeill's, criticise anyone, and sycophantically heaped praise on Nightingale and suggested that she had saved many lives. He left it to his friends Farr and Tulloch to tell her the bad news. She later tried to get Sutherland to say that the death rate did not start to fall until he carried out his sanitary improvements, but he would not do so: 'The mortality at Scutari had fallen off before our Sanitary works – as you will see by the table you have,' he wrote. 'Our works swept the excess away.' That Sutherland should continually 'pull his punches' in this way must have been a source of irritation to her, especially as in the Crimea it had led her into complacency which she would have given anything to avoid. This may have been the unhappiness that underlay her relationship with Sutherland.

The devotion and tolerance shown to Nightingale by close associates like Herbert, Clough, and Sutherland, can be more easily explained by their knowledge of her personal circumstances than any manipulation on her part. With the huge team of people in all walks of life who looked to her for leadership in the cause of social reform, her management methods improved radically after her breakdown. For the rest of her life she adopted an approach that was the extreme opposite of the one she had used during her short hospital management career. She set herself an enormous range of goals after the war. They included making nurses independent of doctors, separating sanitary and medical responsibilities, reducing the use of hospitals in favour of district nurses who would visit homes, modifying accepted standards of hospital architecture, introducing statistical reporting in hospitals, and bringing sanitary engineering expertise into government and local citizens' groups. In addition to these public health questions she became deeply involved in administrative reform and famine relief in India, in education, the relief of poverty, the repeal of legislation unfair to prostitutes, and many other areas. Each of her goals could only be achieved by introducing change at every level of government. During the war she had insisted on being given a title and authority, and had shunned the hospitals where her authority was not well defined. But after the war she never accepted any title or authority at all. No paid official was ever to report to her, and she refused all requests by organisations that wanted to use her name. The fact that she had no official title may have been partly because the title of the post she occupied was not available to a woman: Cabinet Minister without portfolio. As the law did not allow her to stand for parliament, and a Minister must be an MP, such a title was out of the question, but nobody could doubt the justice or democratic legitimacy of her unofficial appointment to the post. If she could have stood for the House of Commons she would have been elected on a landslide. And like other politicians she had the kind of knowledge that was invaluable for securing the cooperation of her Cabinet colleagues: she knew where the bodies were buried.

She lost her youthful desire to enter a competitive profession like a man, and turned against the idea that a woman should have a career. For many years she stopped referring to nursing as a profession, and she opposed the registration of nurses as being the first step in creating a career path. She also naturally opposed the idea of women becoming doctors, a role that better suited the careerist instincts of the male. At Scutari, in her desire to make a career for herself and others, she had micro-managed the nurses' lives; many of them were so oppressed by her tight control that they escaped to other hospitals, a move that she did her utmost to resist. When she began to take an interest in nursing again later in life, her method of controlling nurses was the exact opposite: empowerment.

She monitored probationer nurses' development through written reports from the training school, identified those whom she trusted on the basis of these reports, and then motivated these nurses and ensured that they were given the most important posts. Then she continued to motivate these picked leaders by occasional interviews throughout their career, acting as an employment and information exchange. This hands-off approach to managing nurses may appear to have been chosen by necessity to suit her invalidity. But it is more likely to have been simply a deliberate reversal of her Scutari role, and an endorsement of the view of her friend John Stuart Mill that the 'principal business of the central authority should be to give instruction, the local authority to apply it. Power may be localised, but knowledge to be most useful must be centralised.'

Amy Hughes is an example of a nurse whom Nightingale developed in this way. Hughes trained at St Thomas's in 1885, and as was the custom at the end of her training paid a visit on Nightingale. The Sage of South Street lay on her couch and chatted for a while, then suddenly announced that her visitor was to become a 'district nurse' – attending the sick poor in their homes rather than in hospital. Hughes was startled by this news, but as Nightingale went on to describe the necessity for such work with great feeling, Hughes felt that she had no alternative but to agree even though she had worked for her training and had no obligation to Nightingale or her Fund. Nightingale thereafter interviewed her every year, and twice made her change jobs. After ten years, Nightingale revised Amy Hughes' instruction book for district nurses, introducing much new material including detailed instructions for sterilising milk while retaining its nutrients. It must have been a source of pride to Nightingale that the woman she selected and commanded to help keep the poor away from hospitals should take to it well enough to write an instruction book 'to help my fellow-workers in the service of the poor' as Hughes put it on the title page. As a special mark of favour, Nightingale allowed Hughes to dedicate the book to her 'with permission', although she insisted that Hughes remove a reference to Nightingale's having helped to write it.

A factor which contributed to the disaster in the East had been the failure to use effectively the available means of communication to share information between hospitals and to obtain expert advice. A simple weekly report of deaths sent from her hospital to the military authorities in the Crimea would have saved thousands of lives. Because of this, statistical reporting in hospitals became an obsession of Nightingale's in later life. In addition, she used the Post Office to great effect in maintaining a network of suppliers of public health information. She is thought to have been one of the most prolific letter writers that the world is ever likely to know, rivalling or exceeding Charles Dickens. At least 12,000 of her letters are known to survive and many previously unknown ones come to light each year, often preserved as family heirlooms. The number known or suspected to have been deliberately destroyed is also large. Relatively few of her letters were on family and social business. She maintained a nation-wide network of experts, and ensured the diffusion of their information by putting them in touch with government departments in need of advice and arranging for them to be paid.

The Post Office had stopped charging recipients for the carriage of letters only fifteen years before the Crimean war, when it began subsidising the pre-paid penny post which encouraged the flow of unsolicited information. The Victorian postal system was by the 1860s a marvel of efficiency, and Nightingale exploited it to the full. In a letter to a chemist who developed techniques for measuring the purity of air and water, she requests him to provide a report on water analysis for the War Office and gives him instructions on how to get paid from public funds. The envelope is consigned simply to 'Dr R. Angus Smith Esq. PhD, Manchester' above Nightingale's imperious command 'To be forwarded'. She didn't need to know the address, the Post Office would find it out; Nightingale had discovered the information superhighway. Angus Smith was one of a very few experts whom Nightingale mentioned approvingly by name (twice) in *Notes on Nursing*. He went on to become the country's first salaried environmental protection officer. It is highly unlikely that Nightingale ever met him; he seems to have been typical of the many unassuming and dedicated public servants who benefited from being part of the extensive Nightingale postal network.

Her disability did not interfere with her work, and may well have increased her productivity. She was in regular written communication with hundreds of public health administrators, but hardly saw anyone in person except Sutherland. One notable exception was the Minister who had just been appointed to head the Local Government Board, replacing the old Poor Law Board, who in 1871 was invited to Nightingale's bedside to hear why he should dispense with John Simon's services, which he did.

This was her most intense period of work – those first fifteen years following her recovery from collapse in 1857 at the end of the Royal Commission. The small army of her collaborators was soon whittled down by early death: Sidney Herbert, Alexis Soyer, the reformer of army kitchens, Arthur Clough, and Thomas Alexander, her nominated head of the Army Medical Department. She toiled on, as if seeking a martyrdom of unseen suffering and hard labour like that of the soldiers abandoned by their country during that first terrible winter above Sebastopol.

Nightingale's way of working makes it hard to measure her success by customary standards, and public health is a sensitive and complex enough subject that even modern biographies steer clear of analysing, or even reporting, her disputes with John Simon. There is a revisionist school of thought that claims that in great reform movements a leader with a dominant and ambitious personality usually slows down the spontaneous organic process of reform within society's institutions. Nightingale's rival John Simon is cited as an example of an apparently charismatic leader who was in reality a parasite attached to one such spontaneous process, diverting a small part of its energy to feed his own career ambitions. The rapid improvement of sanitation and medical education in the nineteenth century, for both of which Nightingale worked assiduously behind the scenes, saying 'I am more useful off the stage than on it', are quoted as examples of these organic processes of reform that proceeded more smoothly precisely because they did not have an obvious leader.

CHAPTER EIGHT

Reputation and Myth

Historians agree that Nightingale destroyed part of her correspondence during the years after the war. We might expect that she would do this to protect her reputation, but even her worst critics are surprised that she carefully preserved so much that obviously casts her in a bad light, including evidence of her callous treatment of Sidney Herbert and her jibes at Lord Panmure about whom she later admitted she had been mistaken. It is probably true that she preserved the bad as well as the good as a duty to history, but that does not explain why she *did* destroy some historically important material. A thorough re-examination of the records in the light of her post-war discovery shows that there is a pattern to the destruction. It concerns the discussion of alternative explanations for the deaths at Scutari before she came to accept Farr's diagnosis in May 1857. The most conspicuous example of her censorship is the destruction of correspondence between her and Farr while she was in the process of conversion to his theories during March and April of that year. A letter from William Farr confirmed that he had reluctantly destroyed at her request all the letters she wrote him from that period. In her own file of letters from Farr, now in the British Library, there is no correspondence at all from the period of her conversion between mid-February and early May 1857, while the periods before and after are filled with letters. This shows clearly where the focus of her destruction lay.

In these destroyed letters she must have continued to promote the theory of her friend McNeill that the men were already dying when they entered her hospital. She must have written many other letters before she met Farr, expounding this view that their previous ill-treatment by the army had killed them. She apparently destroyed nearly all such letters, or persuaded their correspondents to destroy them. This is not an assumption that the absence of evidence is itself evidence, because one such letter *did* survive – the one already quoted, which she had written to the War Minister in August 1855: 'The physically deteriorating effect of the Scutari air has been much discussed but it may be doubted. The men sent down to Scutari in the winter died because they were not sent down till half dead – the men sent down now live and recover because they are sent in time.' The letter shows that she did not at that time believe that Sutherland's Sanitary Commission had made any difference to the death rate at Scutari in the spring of 1855. The difference between this letter and the others known to be missing is that this was sent to someone with whom she was not on close enough terms to retrieve it – as she is known to have done with the missing ones.

Her destruction of the correspondence was so comprehensive that we are only able to date her conversion to Farr's theories by noting when the hole appears in her records, and by picking up fragments from around the rim of the crater, so to speak. Another such fragment is the letter that she wrote to McNeill in May 1857, telling him that she had informed Queen Victoria that bad hygiene in her hospitals had killed the soldiers, obviously a new finding. The original of this letter is missing, and we know that she retrieved her letters to McNeill, but her inquisitive sister had made a copy of it which survives.

Nightingale went to extraordinary lengths to track down the originals of letters that she had written during the period when she was, as we would say now, in denial of Farr's theory and just before her breakdown when she finally accepted his conclusion. She persuaded some of her correspondents to destroy them – like Farr – while others returned them to her so that she could selectively destroy them herself. The censorship tended to focus on the correspondence with her closest confidants. Conspicuously missing from the period are letters to her religious adviser Cardinal Manning, to Reverend Mother Mary Clare, her confidante at the Bermondsey Convent, to Colonel Lefroy, to Arthur Clough, and nearly all letters to her family between 13 July and 15 August 1857. In many cases she had to wait until after the recipient's death to recover her letters. Her recovery exercise explains why there are so many original letters from Nightingale in her own papers now in the British library. They include her letters to Sidney Herbert, which she demanded that he return just before her breakdown. On that occasion Herbert replied to his old friend gently and sadly refusing her request: 'I enclose a batch of your papers. But I do not give up my rights of property, our engagement not having been broken off you have no right to have your letters back.' After Herbert died, Nightingale visited his home at Wilton and removed these letters. In those days there was no Cabinet Office for the preservation of Ministerial papers, and Ministers took them home when they left office. That's why the letter that Nightingale wrote to Herbert's successor, in which she claimed that the patients of the first winter were too far gone to recover, survived in the Panmure family archives in Scotland, where she could not retrieve it.

In some cases she appears to have been extremely selective, only destroying parts of letters. For example, one of her letters to Herbert in

March 1857 says 'I now send you some sanitary figures . . .' The rest of the letter is missing. The missing figures may have made reference to Farr's new theory, and her denial of it. The absence of a separate leaf may be accidental, but there is a more significantly incomplete letter to Nightingale from Colonel Lefroy. In it Lefroy begins to discuss the differences in relative mortality in the Crimea and at Scutari, but just as he does so the remainder of the letter is torn off, which cannot be an accident. Lefroy wrote this letter just after Nightingale returned to England, and it is quite possible that the missing pages contained Nightingale's first glimpse of the mortality figures that Tulloch had prepared and then suppressed at the government's request. There may well have been some reference in Lefroy's letter to Nightingale's claim that 'the Scutari air' was not to blame.

Sir Edward Cook, the first biographer to have access to Nightingale's papers after her death, found that she had carefully organised her papers dating from before 1861, and had obviously destroyed many of them. From that date onwards, she seemed to have preserved virtually everything. This also supports the theory that she had something to hide from the early period. The most obvious explanation would be that she wanted to protect her Crimean reputation, but this doesn't fit with the pattern of destruction. If that had been her objective then she could easily have destroyed much more. She could have destroyed the letters that she had written to Lefroy and Herbert from the Crimea in which she was conspicuously silent on the need for improvements to sewers and ventilation. If she had destroyed these letters it would have helped to perpetuate the myth, circulated in her lifetime by Kinglake in his ponderous history of the war, that it was she who had called for the Sanitary Commission to be sent to Scutari. In any case, if she wanted to protect her reputation, why would she print and disseminate against the government's wishes her Confidential Report, *Notes on Matters Affecting the Health of the British Army*, which remains to this day the only known evidence that her hospitals were more than twice as lethal as the hospitals in the Crimea that she had denigrated during the war?

There is one way to explain her very selective destruction of the records: she thought that she was going to die and was worried that after her death some of her letters of criticism of Farr and defence of her hospital could be used by the enemies of sanitary reform to discredit Farr and challenge his theories. This is borne out by the evidence cited by Zachary Cope that she asked Farr to destroy her letters in connection with her supposed imminent death. The destruction is that of a woman concerned with a purely operational matter: the successful implementation of sanitary reforms. She could not allow her death to interfere with her purpose.

An indicator of how she viewed her own reputation is that after the spring of 1857, when Nightingale completed her statistical analysis with Farr, she never spoke of her mission at Scutari in favourable terms. This is

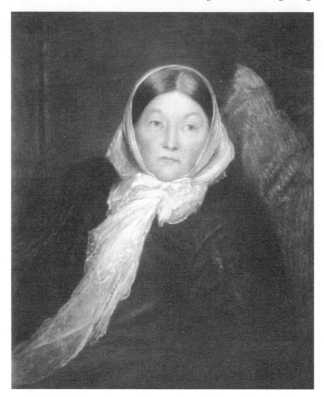

Florence Nightingale
in 1887.

in marked contrast to the period before that date, when she was sometimes quite vainglorious about it. One illustration of her later reluctance to express satisfaction with her work at Scutari is in a letter she wrote to her aunt in August 1887 containing a rare retrospective self-congratulation. She conspicuously omits to mention the value of her work up to her breakdown, including her war service and the Royal Commission: 'In this month 34 years ago you lodged me in Harley Street. And in this month, 31 years ago you returned me to England from Scutari. And in this month 30 years ago the first Royal Commission was finished. And since then, 30 years of work often cut to pieces but never destroyed.' She could easily have written, 'In all, 34 years of work often cut to pieces . . .' Such omissions are admittedly very inconclusive, and neither Nightingale nor any of the people closest to her are known to have left any reminiscences confirming that she blamed herself for the failures during the war. Nightingale may not have known, may not have admitted that her feelings of guilt were even important to her. But Farr, Herbert, Tulloch, McNeill, Lefroy, Sutherland, and others could not have failed to understand the reason for her obsessive activity, her moods, and her attacks on her family. Some of them must have felt at least partly responsible for the official blunders that had given her so much responsibility and had led her into a personal disaster. They surrounded her like a bodyguard: tolerant to her whims, impervious to her insults and sarcasm, discreetly carrying out her nagging orders to the letter, and taking her secrets to the grave.

But Nightingale would not be Nightingale if she couldn't find a way to leave behind some trace of her feelings without having to acknowledge them. The obvious places to look for a leakage of her emotions would be in her mystical writings, particularly the collection entitled *Suggestions for Thought*, which she wrote in the months following her breakdown. This was an expanded version, running to 800 pages, of a sixty-nine page work that she had printed in 1852, before she went to the war. She began to write *Suggestions for Thought* as a description of the religious doubts that she attributed to ordinary people, and her answers to them. It started life in 1852 under the title *To the Artizans of England*, her response to some cynical arguments put to her by working-class men in the villages surrounding her father's estate in Derbyshire. Indignant, and perhaps unable to counter their arguments face to face, she had laboured earnestly over a pamphlet which rebutted their atheistical views. After the war, this pamphlet in its expanded version became *Suggestions for Thought to the Searchers after Truth among the Artizans of England*. Then in its

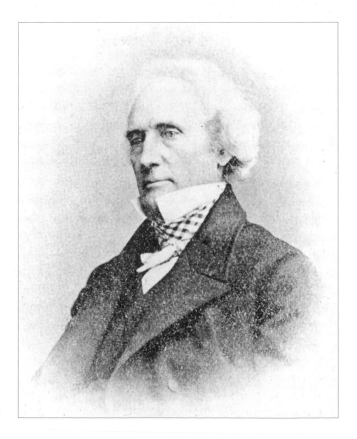

Sir John McNeill in 1866.

final volume the audience was no longer the artisans; the title became *Suggestions for Thought to Searchers after Religious Truth*.

Who had these searchers become in 1860, if they were no longer the artisans of 1852? Was there now only one searcher after religious truth, and was her name Florence Nightingale? The 1860 version of this book (of which only six printed copies are known to have existed) was only seen by her closest confidants. Her mentor, former mutual worshipper and still close friend Sir John McNeill, who knew better than anyone what she had been through, was one of them. McNeill pronounced the work totally unsuited for the purpose for which she said it was intended: the conversion of unbelievers. However, he added the enigmatic prediction that it was a 'mine from which one day much precious metal may be drawn.' Such a work should indeed be a goldmine of personal information, because of her claim that it contains her spiritual guidance to a public suffering from religious doubts. When people are feeling an emotion that they are unwilling or unable to admit they are often very ready to attribute it to others, in the phenomenon of *projection*. A psychologist can often explore a subject's innermost feelings by giving her an opportunity to make speculative generalisations about other people's feelings.

Suggestions for Thought is a collection of oblique suggestions of things that Florence Nightingale ought to start thinking about without fear. Things like guilt, remorse, suffering and evil. It could be subtitled: *Notes on Matters Affecting the Mind of Miss Florence Nightingale, Founded on the Experience of the Russian War*. Virtually everything that is in the 1852 version of her religious testament survives in slightly altered form in the 1860 *Suggestions for Thought*. A comparison of the two documents allows us to study the continuity and change in Nightingale's most private thinking before and after the war and, more important, after her post-war discoveries.

The 1852 version was a rather dry and theoretical proof that human nature is innately good despite the fact that the historical record seems to show the contrary. Nightingale claimed that our recognition of past evil is in itself proof that we can avoid it in future. Human progress will occur purely as a result of our innate ability to recognise evil. Sinners do not need to feel remorse, neither is there any need for God to punish them. What we must do is strive to improve our ability to distinguish good from evil.

The Nightingale philosophy had no room in it for distinctions between sin, ignorance, evil, mistakes, and crime. These were all the result of the perpetrators' failure to understand cause and effect relationships. Knowledge of God's laws would eventually abolish all of them. Those who make mistakes, she said, are the pioneers: 'The pioneer's is the highest calling, and God calls the highest men to it. But thieves and murderers, who are also His calling, are in some sense His pioneers!' During the war she had told Lord Raglan proudly that 'My father's religious and social ethics make us strive to be the pioneers of the human race.' When she did so she was already including herself in a category that contained thieves and murderers, because she had already defined it thus in the 1852 version of her tract. This gives some idea of the broad-minded philosophy with which her father had equipped her. Oddly, the 1852 version also mentions 'sanitary science', but in its older sense of medical care rather than drainage. She used it in 1852 to argue that minds can be made healthy by following good religious advice in the same way that the body can benefit physically from 'sanitary science' i.e. medical counsel.

One of the most remarkable aspects of Nightingale's thought is that many of her concepts, including the religious ones, survived the shocks of the war and its aftermath. After she found out about her failure at Scutari, we might have expected her to conclude that it had been juvenile arrogance that had dared to disguise itself as the voice of God calling her to work in hospitals. We might have expected her to remark that calls from God are a sign of over-confidence coupled with a lack of basic training. But many private notes show that her faith was unchanged, and God continued to speak to her. Likewise, her belief in the perfectibility of man and the duty of mankind to strive for perfection, was a cornerstone of her beliefs after the war as it had been before. The post-war *Suggestions for Thought* confirms this.

To say that these mental constructions survived intact is only another way of saying that they helped her to survive a shock that would have driven many over the brink. It is to acknowledge that the conceptual framework with which she started was of a strong manufacture. One of the concepts that was to stand her in good stead was that of using numeric data to support proposals for social change. We have seen that unfortunately she was not familiar before the war with Farr's use of death statistics in public health. She was, however, familiar with the use of statistics in social science, pioneered by Adolphe Quetelet. Even before the war she was fascinated by Quetelet's work. She went considerably further than him in her belief that statistics, by revealing cause and effect relationships which were not visible at the level of the individual, could help administrators to improve society. This belief is at the root of the optimistic advice in her *Suggestions for Thought*. She was much more optimistic than Quetelet himself, who thought that the main benefit of his discoveries would be intellectual satisfaction.

One reason that British followers like Nightingale could be more optimistic about the practical application of Quetelet's theories was that in Britain the industrial revolution had given them practical experience of how numerical approaches could help to increase productivity. Jeremy Bentham's 'greatest happiness for the greatest number' was an attempt to apply the concepts of industrial revolution to social issues, much to the distress of some humanists who found it inappropriate to count human happiness like ingots of pig iron. Edwin Chadwick had begun his career as Bentham's protégé, and Chadwick's unfeeling reliance on numbers and productivity was part of the reason for his inability to mobilise public opinion. After her breakdown, Nightingale's softer approach and her emotional commitment helped to free the sanitarian movement from Chadwick's utilitarian taint.

Nightingale adapted Quetelet's theories to make them more practical and more acceptable to philanthropists. Quetelet's demonstration that statistical methods could predict accurately even something as capricious as the number of twenty-year-old men marrying sixty-year-old women, or the number of murders committed with each type of weapon, made it appear that free will was less important than many philanthropists would like. Nightingale met this problem head on by denying the importance of free will at the individual level, even contradicting Quetelet. In the absence of knowledge, she claimed, the ability of the individual to choose was limited, and in the presence of knowledge any rational being would make the same choice. She wrote in *Suggestions for Thought* how unimportant her supposed 'free will' had been in determining her own actions: 'Could I, when I knew the soldiers were being murdered wholesale, decide otherwise than to give all I had to prevent it?' This was a revealingly ambiguous rhetorical question. Was she referring to the murdered soldiers at Scutari, or to the 1,200 soldiers a year who she found afterwards were being killed by defective sanitation in their barracks in England? In both cases her free will had been the same but the statistical information at her disposal was different and, therefore, so were her actions.

Nightingale came to believe that Quetelet had discovered in statistics the language that God uses for telling us what to do in order to improve mankind. Quetelet had in fact discovered an empirical proof that 'we are members one of another' – each of us is a variation on a theme, something that was by no means understood before. This enables us to use empirical data to predict the effect on society of an administrator's actions. She wrote of 'the application of Quetelet's discoveries to explaining the plan of God in teaching us by these results the laws of progress – to explaining the path on which we must go if we are to discover the laws of the Divine Government'. She used the word 'law' almost as a synonym for cause and effect relationship. The world is made up of these causes and effects but they are only gradually being identified by mankind. according to her. The most powerful tool for doing so is the statistical method, which arrays apparently unrelated facts in such a way as to allow man to relate the cause to the effect. The reason that she may have used the term 'law' instead of talking of cause and effect is that in her Unitarian way she did not like the word 'cause', as it invited a lot of useless theorising of the kind the medical profession or the Church indulged in; statistical evidence was more important.

God requires us, therefore, to work by trial and error. Statistics only work after the fact. To learn how to prevent premature death, many such deaths must occur in a controlled environment and someone must wish to make use of the experience gained. That, she now knew, was why God had called her. This optimistic analysis was the positive side *of Suggestions for Thought,* the logical part, the thoughts that she attributes to herself as writer of the book. The book also describes some negative, more emotional, thoughts. These she attributes to the 'other', the reader, the 'searcher after religious truth' whom she was trying to help by writing these suggestions. Nightingale's philosophy as expounded in the book will, she hopes, help to drive these bad thoughts out of the reader's mind. The bad thoughts, on examination, turn out to be what one would expect of a well-meaning woman who is tortured by the discovery of her ignorant participation in a slaughter of the innocents.

In her book, Nightingale tells the tormented searcher after religious truth that she should not feel remorse and guilt for past mistakes because these mistakes were a part of God's plan. Nightingale assures the searcher that evil is necessary in God's scheme to achieve perfection, and that in feeling remorse and guilt the searcher is actually obstructing His plan because these negative feelings prevent her from concentrating on the tasks He has given her. If the searcher after truth is experiencing guilt she must realise that there will be no forgiveness for her and other criminals because God believes that forgiveness is not only unnecessary but would also be unkind. Throughout the book, Nightingale uses the plural 'we' to express her 'official' beliefs: the optimistic philosophy that she claims to have and that she wishes the reader to adopt. Occasionally, an 'I' appears, usually when expressing a bad thought which needs correcting, as if to get closer to the reader by imagining the reader's individual situation. An example is the following description of counterproductive guilt. There is a sudden change from 'our' to 'I' in the first sentence and then the closer to her guilt she comes, the more confused the personal pronouns, as Nightingale loses her selves in a hall of verbal mirrors and shifting identities:

Our belief amounts to this: that I may look back on any particular moment of the past, and truly feel that it was impossible at that moment (God's laws being what they are, and having operated on all preceding that moment as they did) that I should have willed other than as I did. It is therefore untrue and useless for me to cry out 'Oh, how worthy of blame, how deserving of punishment I was.' My good friend, I should rather say to myself 'don't be afraid, you will have suffering enough in what you have done. You exhaust the powers which you have in you for finding out the laws to alter nature or circumstance, by these exclamations.' 'Come back,' I would say kindly to myself, 'I know you could not help it. Let us have patience with ourself, and see what we can do.'

The cure for remorse, according to Nightingale, is extremely simple: it is to realise that it does not exist. 'Remorse is not a true feeling – not a feeling of what really is; for remorse is blame to ourselves for the past. But if the origin of our will, and our will itself, were, as it has been, in accordance with law, there cannot in truth be blame to ourselves personally, individually.'

While advising the searcher after truth not to waste time on remorse, Nightingale uses the official 'our', but does go so far as to admit to having strayed down the forbidden path of remorse herself. 'Our experience is, that to dwell on the past error with feelings of remorse depresses the energy, all of which is wanted to pursue the right in future.' This admission that the writer has personal 'experience' of remorse was added after the war. In her earlier 1852 tract we find word for word the quotations above about remorse 'not being a true feeling', one which distracts people from good works. The difference is that in 1852 there is never any mention that the writer might ever have experienced it. No cry from the heart 'Oh, how worthy of blame, how deserving of punishment I was'; no admission that the author has herself been guilty of the sin of remorse. A sentence in the 1860 version: 'To look back on my life is to look back upon a tissue of mistakes,' was not present in 1852.

One reason why remorse is not a 'true feeling' is that God himself is the author of all the evil for which men may blame themselves: 'God's laws are the origin of moral, as of physical evil – that it is so is part of His righteous rule. Through them, by our mistakes, we find truth; by our errors, knowledge; by our sufferings, happiness; by our evil, good.' In 1852, mankind had to learn how to recognise evil. It was no good relying on remorse to identify evil that we have done, as we have seen, and it was no good thinking God was going to punish us, for example by visiting cholera upon us as was vulgarly supposed. God is more merciful than that. God has given us an innate ability to recognise good and evil so He does not need to use punishments as a deterrent. But in 1860 there is a major departure on this point from the 1852 version. During that interval she has discovered that God does need to use punishment after all: 'We find that [i.e. an official Nightingale belief follows] *punishment*, if the word be used in the sense of suffering or privation consequent on sin or ignorance, does exist in God's moral government, and we see it to be right, because its effect will be sooner or later to induce mankind to remedy the evils which incur it.'

Remorse is still not true, but suffering God's punishment for mistakes has now become essential to the learning process. Nightingale seems to have made this fine distinction to disguise the internal nature of her afflictions. She could not admit that her suffering was the result of her own emotional distress. God is, in 1860, inflexible in His punishment, and fortunately is not prone to 'having mercy on His erring children. This mercy would be the height of cruelty. As long as His laws have not inflicted evil consequences on our sin and ignorance till no vestige of either is left in us, mercy means to leave us in sin and consequently in misery.' Punishment can only be useful when applied to the living. Eternal damnation cannot possibly exist, says Nightingale, because it would not be a remedial punishment. It would not serve God's purpose of promoting human progress.

All sin, says Nightingale, arises from ignorance of God's laws. By law, as we have already seen, Nightingale meant something like a cause and effect relationship. Because mankind can, by examination of statistics, learn how these laws operate, he can ensure that evil is only 'temporary', i.e. does not affect all future generations. Like a good teacher, God gives us an eternity to solve each of our problems. In this eternity there will always remain some evil unresolved, but 'there will not be always masses of evil, lying untouched, unpenetrated by light and wisdom'. The most important addition to the philosophy in 1860 is an explanation of how philanthropists could cause new evils by their ignorant intervention, and yet still be doing God's work: 'Each advance has always brought evil with good, because each advance must, in some degree, be made upon a hypothesis. But mankind, because men are similar to each other, will more and more speedily turn the evil into good . . . there will be a perpetual and rapid change of evil into good; thence fresh temporary evil, thence fresh permanent good.'

As an example of man-made evil she quoted Quetelet's finding that charities which took in abandoned children increased child mortality dramatically by encouraging mothers to abandon them in unhealthy crowded institutions. Although inevitable, such philanthropic evil would be easy to remedy due to the philanthropists' skill at identifying and rectifying their own mistakes. This also explained, of course, why the disaster at Scutari should lead to rapid improvements in public health that more than compensated for it.

It may not be too surprising, against this background of the sufferings identified in *Suggestions for Thought*, that Nightingale appeared to identify herself with Christ. Or, it might be more accurate to say that she may have believed that Christ had a similar problem to hers. She dismissed outright the possibility that God might have made Christ suffer for the sins of others – that did not fit in with her scheme of improvement at all. The implication is that Christ suffered for a mistake of his own. Nightingale talked about Christ in a familiar way, as if she thought that she understood him as a human being, and it may be that she imagined that he, too, had been one of God's pioneers: 'Christ's whole life almost was a war upon the family,' she wrote approvingly. She thought him a 'beautiful tender spirit' but criticised his rather off-hand attitude to public health, morals, and education. Some of her private religious writings have caused embarrassment because they seem to equate her sufferings with Christ's, as in the following note written in about 1868:

> I have seen his face. The crown of glory inseparably united with the Crown of Thorns giving forth the same light. Three times he has called me. Once to his service Feb 7 1837. Once to be a Deliverer May 7 1852. Once to the cross July 28 1865 to suffer more even that I have hitherto done aut pati aut mori [either to suffer or to die] for on the Cross I shall see his face. Am I being offered to him? Then this is his answer. The crown of thorns round the light and radiant head. And is it not worth all to see his face? And may I think that I am another Himself, another like that? Oh too happy aut pati aut mori. Oh too blessed that He should look upon me as another like that another in état de victime [made a victim] for all perfection is in that.

In another note she refers to God's call to her to be a 'saviour' on May 7 1852, showing that this word was synonymous with 'deliverer'. It will be remembered that she referred to Colonel Tulloch as a deliverer, and rated McNeill even higher, for their efforts to feed the starving troops in the Crimea. She defines a saviour or deliverer as 'one who saves from social, from moral error' by finding out one or more of the laws of God. It is not clear whether she had a theory to explain how Christ earned the status of saviour, and the right to suffer. In her philosophy a person could suffer for her sins for her whole lifetime, but no suffering was to be eternal and she did not seem to believe in heaven. She thought that the dead sufferer would be allowed to participate in, and experience the lives of future, less suffering generations – a state that she called 'continued identity'. This was in tune with her own consuming interest in the long-term improvement of society and her disdain for the pursuit of short-term individual goals.

She did not foresee a heavenly park for disembodied spirits but rather a future existence in which the dead could continue to exercise their full range of individual and idiosyncratic human capabilities. Mere communication between the dead and the living would not be sufficient relief for the departed sinners who had suffered so much in their lifetime. Justice would require that they should be able to actively participate after their death in the better life on earth that they helped to create. 'Without the belief in a continued identity, there is really no belief in [God's] wise and good superintendence,' she confessed. 'What would we say of a Being who could cause such sufferings for no future benefit to the sufferer, but for future temporary benefit to some future being?' The continued identity theme is one that only appeared after the war, in the 1860 version of *Suggestions for Thought*. It seems that she was hoping for some sort of multiple reincarnation into the personalities of later identities. She could presumably help to make this come true, for herself, by devoting all her idiosyncratic individual capabilities in life to the pursuit and promotion of goals that would create those future identities.

If Nightingale planned to live on in future generations, it was not her intention to do so through her public reputation. This is fortunate because the distortion of her reputation that took place after her death was truly astonishing. An examination of the information sources available shows that during her lifetime many people must have known that the sentimental wartime propaganda portrait of her was embarrassingly false. Even Kinglake, when he alleged in 1880 that she was responsible for the creation of the Crimean Sanitary Commission, did so in terms that seemed to admit that he had no real evidence: he simply says that the commission's instructions betrayed the hand of a woman! After her death, various self-seeking organisations and individuals dusted off her old wartime image and added a varnish of new myths about her role in the training of modern hospital nurses. The 1911 *Dictionary of National Biography* seized on Kinglake's half-hearted claim and dressed it up, saying that only 'after Miss Nightingale's persistent entreaties' did the government send out the Sanitary Commission. This remained the official view until the *Dictionary* was rewritten in 2004.

A very large number of educated people after 1857 knew of Nightingale's theory that her hospital had caused a disproportionate number of the fatalities during the war. Many influential people in all walks of life had received private copies of her confidential report pointing out how the mortality 'was due to the frightful state of the Hospitals at Scutari; how much it depended on the number which each Regiment was unfortunately enabled to send to those pest-houses'. This allegation appeared in the first few pages, and in an annex there was also a table of data to support it. Five hundred copies of the report went to the most influential citizens in the country. The recipients must have talked of it with others but obeyed the strict instructions that she gave them not to publish it, leave it lying around, or refer to it in writing. From letters of the time it appears that in those days people could make sensational revelations in confidence to their correspondents under the simple admonition that the revelations were 'private'. People could be trusted, but nevertheless it must be assumed that the revelations in the 'confidential report' leaked to a very wide audience by word of mouth, though never in print. Most medical people would also know that she had changed her mind during the Royal Commission, because she had widely canvassed her old theory in letters that she later retrieved and destroyed.

We cannot so easily guess what might have been the opinions of the mass of the population. Was she always to them simply the merciful angel of Scutari, whose personal purity had silenced the curses in the soldiers' throats and made the rough surgeons gentle? Is it only because of our own supposedly superior modern intellect that the 'real' Florence Nightingale is now emerging? Strangely enough it is possible that between 1857 and 1910 the whole country knew much more about Nightingale's remorse and her personal problems than did later generations. The Nightingale myth may be a modern reinvention.

People who were not chosen to receive her confidential report must have heard the inside story from those 'in authority' who were. In addition, some popular books powerfully criticising Nightingale appeared during and just after the war from nurses who had worked under her. An example is Mrs Davis's 1857 autobiography, which in an appendix contains the allegation that Nightingale's own 'Barrack Hospital at Scutari continued to present the greatest amount of least alleviated misery of any war hospital belonging to the British Army of the East.' More importantly, Nightingale herself ensured that the mass of the population received information that would counter the wartime propaganda. One of the people to whom she sent her confidential report was Harriet Martineau, a famous and successful popular journalist of the time. They agreed that Martineau would do a series of articles and a book, which Nightingale wanted to be published very cheaply to get wide circulation. She volunteered to pay Martineau to write the book, eventually called *England and her Soldiers*.

Nightingale stipulated that Martineau must base the work on extracts from public documents, even though she could use the confidential report for additional background information. (The main difference between the public and confidential documents was the latter's condemnation of Nightingale's own hospital). Martineau must also not attribute any information to Nightingale and Nightingale insisted on revising the proofs, 'to guard against "innocent mistakes" as you say.' The phrase shows that they both knew it was censorship. Nightingale did change the proofs – she made Martineau include additional material about military tactics so that there could be a pretext for putting the book in regimental libraries. She told Martineau she hoped to arrange this with the help of Colonel Lefroy who had been given the job of founding the Army Educational Corps, though Lefroy's absence for two months at the critical time interfered with this plan. The book stated that thousands of soldiers had been killed in hospital due to bad ventilation, and that Nightingale's own Barrack Hospital had been the worst-ventilated of all. On the few occasions when the book mentions Nightingale, it describes her as a helpless participant rather than as a monumental figure for whom the hospital might have been designed as a stage on which to exhibit her greatness. She is shown attending to the personal cleanliness of the victims and 'preparing them for surgery' – one of the recurring nightmares of families must have been the idea that their loved ones died in agony under the amputation saw. No soldiers were described kissing anybody's shadow, or anything remotely similar. There was no indication that Nightingale had anything to do with the book's production.

Martineau sent a copy of *England and her Soldiers* to Sidney Herbert, recently returned as Minister of War. She suggested to Herbert it would be a good idea to put a copy in each regimental library. Herbert was not sympathetic to the idea. 'It is a book for the authorities rather than for the men' he told her. When Nightingale's friend Lefroy returned, Nightingale tried to get him to approve the army library scheme, but Lefroy said that he could not go against the decision of his chief. Nightingale thereupon donated her own fifty copies to the lending libraries in 'Mechanics Institutes' throughout the country. There it would be read by the same 'artisans of England' with whom she had discussed her optimistic religious theories before the war. *England and her Soldiers* must have had a relatively large popular readership; it was perhaps of more interest to civilian members of Mechanics Institutes, whose sons had died in the hospitals, than it would have been to soldiers, and must have gained wide readership and publicity for the revelation that the Barrack Hospital had been the worst of all.

By the time the book was published in 1859, Nightingale had not been seen or heard of for a while. The contrast between her and Mary Seacole was striking. Seacole was the heroic entrepreneurial nurse who ran her own convivial hotel at the front and clambered over the battlefields with a satchel of bandages. On her return to England, Seacole openly wore the Crimea Medal, a departure from the rules that was apparently tolerated by the authorities. Lord Palmerston tried to award Nightingale a medal too, and she was certainly more entitled to one than Seacole, having been in the Crimea with an official title and on army business. No record remains of Nightingale's reaction to Palmerston's proposal, but we can assume it would have been negative. Immediately after the war, Seacole was sporting her Crimea Medal proudly and living the high life in London, deservedly feted by the war's veterans and publishing to wide acclaim her account of her exploits. But where was Miss Florence Nightingale? She was not recounting her experiences as a lesson to the nation's youth, or basking with Mother Seacole on the music-hall stage. She was in hiding. Martineau's book and Nightingale's disappearance must have changed the general public's perception of Nightingale and her work at Scutari. So must the publication of her strange and very popular *Notes on Nursing* in early 1860. Perhaps it will never be possible to tell how much the mass of the population knew of the truth about Florence Nightingale between 1860 and 1900. It seems unlikely that the image of the angel of Scutari survived intact, although whenever her name was mentioned in public there were cheers.

Starting in the early 1880s, the middle-aged Nightingale appeared to regain some serenity and happiness, and became more physically mobile. She even went on holiday to the seaside for several weeks, and once visited St Thomas's Hospital. She started to take an interest in the Nightingale Training School, and formed sentimental attachments with some of the more able nurses there. She became very close to her sister and to Parthe's husband and step-children, and often stayed with them. Perhaps she gained some insight into the real reason for the personal unhappiness that she had previously blamed on her family. More likely she had become aware that the very high mortality from the most destructive epidemic fevers, which her rival John Simon had called unavoidable, had been falling sharply for some years. This would have cheered her.

By the time Nightingale died in 1910, aged ninety, none of her contemporaries remained to contradict any posthumous distortions of her memory. The significance of her confidential report and the reasons for its suppression had been forgotten. Many of the copies she distributed found their way into medical collections, where the annex containing the secret of Scutari lay unremarked for more than a century like the time capsule that she must have intended. Her family destroyed some of the huge volume of papers that Nightingale left behind because they were too controversial, and paid Sir Edward Cook to write a biography that would emphasise the role of the Nightingale Training School, in which they had a interest. Cook was a warmongering journalist and an active participant in the tightening of government censorship before and during the First World War, and he carefully covered up Nightingale's conflicts with the authorities and her whistleblowing.

In the 1940s, a later generation of Nightingale's family asked Mrs Woodham-Smith to write a new biography that would expose family conflicts, which an earlier generation had forbidden Cook to describe and which fascinated 1950s England so much. In emphasising this aspect, Woodham-Smith promoted a theory that Nightingale's breakdown was caused by her relationship with her mother and sister. Woodham-Smith borrowed political and nursing material from Cook and thus inadvertently perpetuated his censorship of Nightingale's conflicts with Queen Victoria and with John Simon, the national Chief Medical Officer, and exaggerated Nightingale's post-war involvement in the Training School.

The tendency of biographers to rely almost exclusively on Nightingale's own archives has also obscured some of the political storms that raged around her and of which, before her shipwreck, she was unaware. The result of the accumulated censorship and family bias was that Nightingale emerged as a highly irrational creature. For example, her struggle over sanitation after the war, when she had supposedly solved the problem without resistance at Scutari, made it seem that she was kicking down an open door. Nightingale, by herself destroying the evidence of her conversion for tactical reasons, deepened the mystery. Her twentieth-century biographers did not pay much attention to the claims in her leaked Confidential Report that her hospitals had killed thousands of patients during the months after her arrival. There was probably an understandable reluctance to examine so macabre a claim. What useful purpose could it serve?

In asking whether it serves a useful purpose now, we should ask how Nightingale would have wanted history to remember her. She was contemptuous of the notion that Sidney Herbert would have wanted to be remembered for saving lives. If she was sincere, she would not want to be remembered for this either. Would she then prefer to be forgotten, satisfied simply to achieve her ambition of merging her soul with those of future generations? If this were true, it would be unkind to rake over these old stories. But if it were true she would not have hoarded for posterity the huge archives that give such a fascinating insight into her age, and would not have altered her will later in life to demand their preservation. Nor would she have guaranteed the survival of the officially suppressed evidence of the disaster at Scutari by leaking it.

If she did not want that old discarded individual identity named Florence Nightingale to be remembered for the good that she accomplished, what reputation did she want to emerge from her archive? She always maintained that the sentimental reputation for her achievements at Scutari was the greatest hindrance in her work, because it obscured the lesson that she learned from the Scutari disaster and which she desperately wanted to publicise. When she finally saw that the lesson had paid off she may have wanted to preserve in her archive an example of how 'fresh temporary evil' created by the mistakes of a philanthropist can lead to 'fresh permanent good'. It would be a story of a great blunder by someone whose intentions were above reproach. It doesn't seem such a bad thing to go down in history for. How else might she be remembered if not for that? As a tyrannical invalid? A neurotic meddler in government affairs? As the founder of modern secular nursing, whose right to the title is subject to perpetual scholarly dispute? As a case of brucellosis? Or as – perish the thought – the Lady with the Lamp?

It seems that she may have wanted history to remember how an ambitious young woman responded to a unique opportunity. How her country called on Florence Nightingale in a great national emergency, and sent her with unlimited power and resources to care for the health of 'the finest army that ever left these shores.' To remind us of the lesson learned, she may have wanted history to remember how, through her ignorance and arrogance, she let that army die.

Differences

Some recent published literature on Nightingale disagrees with the interpretation given here. Many of the disagreements arise from a few common errors of fact, which are often traceable to previous historians who may not have had access to crucial documents.

It is a mistake of fact to say that Nightingale was already obsessed with failure when she returned from the Crimean War. Newly discovered documents quoted in my 1998 book show that she wrote proudly of her achievements in the autumn of 1855 and at the end of the war. The mistaken assertion was first made by Woodham-Smith, who relied entirely on an undated note to support it. This note is now known to date from six months after the war and the content makes it clear that it was the discovery of new statistics that caused the gloomy sentiments in it. The mistake helped to support Woodham-Smith's argument that Nightingale was irrational. It was repeated by Young, who used Woodham-Smith as his source. The mistake is commonly repeated today to support the idea that Nightingale's wartime fever caused chronic depression.

It is a more recent error of fact to say that Young's 1995 paper on brucellosis attributed Nightingale's 'depression, with feelings of worthlessness and failure' to her brucellosis. Young only sought an explanation for her physical symptoms to contradict others who attributed them to malingering or psychosomatic causes. Careful reading of his paper shows that he made no attempt to diagnose her 'depression', and his medical references make clear that he could not have attributed it to brucellosis. It is a further error of fact to claim that depression could produce and excuse irritable, cruel, reproachful or tyrannical behaviour.

It is frequently emphasised, erroneously, that Nightingale was only the Superintendent of female nurses at Scutari. None of the literature making this claim quotes the evidence published in Goldie's collection of letters that Herbert had given her additional more reaching responsibilities as a trouble-shooter. It is clear from her actions that Nightingale discharged these additional functions.

Lastly, it has long been said in error that in July 1857 Nightingale finally fixed the blame for Scutari on Sir John Hall. This very important error is based on an incorrect reading of her letter to McNeill in which she referred to the culprit only as 'he'. In 1998, I first published her letter to Herbert of the same date in which she repeated her accusations and directed them at 'you', showing clearly that 'he' in her letter to McNeill was a reference to Herbert. Previously, before she became better-informed, she had indeed blamed Hall, but her correspondence clearly indicates how and why her opinion changed.

Sources

I have not reprinted here the footnotes and bibliography that were included in *Florence Nightingale, Avenging Angel* (Constable, 1998) or in my book *The Crimean War* (Tempus, 2007). Those books are comprehensively indexed and referenced and can be used as references. Where possible I have mentioned new sources in the text of the present book, but in the following cases it was not convenient to do so:

Chapter 1: Ambition.
The evidence that Herbert knew of Nightingale's alleged heresy is quoted in Baly, *Florence Nightingale and the Nursing Legacy* (1997).

Chapter 2: At War.
The more detailed political background relating to McNeill's Supplies Commission can be found in *Florence Nightingale, Avenging Angel*. I have omitted most of it here as being peripheral to Nightingale's story.

Chapter 3: Stirring Events, Romantic Dangers
The letter in which Bracebridge refers to McNeill's 'great fancy' for Nightingale is in bundle 93 in the Clayton archives.

Chapter 4: Post-Mortem
Tulloch's letter of protest to McNeill over the latter's praise of Nightingale is in the National Archives of Scotland, ref. GD371/253/8.

Chapter 5: Conversion
The letter referring to the persecution of McNeill and Tulloch is to Baron Bunsen, 14 February 1857 (Lynn McDonald collection).

Chapter 6: Cover-Up.
The fact that the Sanitary Commission broke 400 windows on their second day comes from *The Times*, 16 October 1858, quoting Rawlinson.

The incident when the Coldstream Guards Colonel went to Scutari to look for his men is described in Wyatt's *History of the First Battalion, Coldstream Guards*, (1858). Hall's statement about avoiding sending patients to Scutari is in his *Observations on the Report of the Sanitary Commissioners* (1857).

The letter referring to 'manslaughter' is to McNeill 24 October 1856 (Copy in Wellcome Institute 8997/9).

The letter about the 'horrid spectre' of Scutari is to Haldane Turriff, 22 April 1869, BL Add. MSS 47757 f107.

Chapter 7: 'By pestilence perished before their time'.
The fallacious theory of Nightingale's opposition to germ theory has now been comprehensively laid to rest by Mark Bostridge and Lynn McDonald and I have not dealt with it again here. I would refer the interested reader to the debate in the *London Review of Books* in December 2008 and January 2009 between those two scholars and Prof. Hugh Pennington.

A book which explores the effectiveness of grass-roots health awareness of the type promoted by Nightingale in *Notes on Nursing* and elsewhere is *The Gospel of Health*, by Nancy Tomes (1998).

For the sidelining of Sir John Simon by Chadwick and Nightingale see Royston Lambert's biography of Simon.

A good commentary on Thomas McKeown's analysis of historical life expectancy can be found in an article by Emily Grundy in the *International Journal of Epidemiology* at *http://ije.oxfordjournals.org/cgi/content/full/34/3/529*

The bipolar disorder theory of Nightingale's illness is to be found in *Post Mortem* by Philip Mackowiak (2007).

Index

Afghanistan, 46
Albert, Prince, 21, 40, 63
Alexander, Thomas, Dr, 135
Alma (battle), 22, 57, 107
Amerian Civil War, 98
Artizans of England (pamphlet), 18, 141
Athena (owlet), 37, 128

Balaclava, 24, 25, 31, 32, 42, 43, 44, 45, 53, 55, 57, 76, 83, 84, 96, 107, 127, 130
Benn, Tony, 13
Bentham, Jeremy, 143
Bermondsey Convent, 56, 138
bipolar disorder, 125, 157
Bostridge, Mark (biographer), 157
Bracebridge, Mr, 48, 49, 50, 63, 156
Bracebridge, Mrs, 34, 36
brucellosis, 48, 53, 123, 124, 131, 153, 154
Burlington Hotel, 10, 64, 72, 102, 103, 123

Cambridge, Duke of, 62, 64
Cassandra, 14, 15
Chadwick, Edwin, 74, 75, 76, 77, 78, 80, 85, 89, 93, 110, 111, 112, 113, 114, 116, 118, 144, 157
Charge of the Light Brigade, 88, 107
cholera, 18, 36, 69, 72, 75, 106, 107, 109, 119, 122, 146
Clough, Arthur, 93, 95, 96, 127, 135, 138

Clough, Martha, 32
Commissariat, 41, 44, 60, 61
confidential report (by Nightingale, 1857-58), 63, 64, 69, 80, 83, 84, 85, 89, 92, 93, 94, 96, 97, 98, 115, 128, 139, 149, 150, 152
Contribution to the Sanitary History ..., 113, 120, 128
Cook, Sir Edward (biographer), 139, 152
Cope, Zachary, 139
coxcomb (diagram), 113, 114, 128
Crimean War, 21, 22

Darwin, Charles, 73, 126
Davis, Elizabeth, 31, 32, 43, 44, 100, 150
depression, 124, 125, 154
diaries, lost, 13
dreaming, 12, 15

Embley Park, 10, 11, 16
entail, law of, 14
Evans, General Sir George de Lacy, 41

Farr, William, 66, 67, 68, 69, 72, 73, 74, 78, 79, 80, 81, 82, 83, 84, 85, 88, 90, 93, 96, 97, 98, 99, 100, 101, 110, 111, 115, 117, 122, 123, 126, 129, 132, 137, 138, 139, 140, 143

Garibaldi, 13
Gavin, Dr Hector, 42, 77, 78

Gill, Gillian (biographer), 11, 15, 16
Gladstone, William, 110, 129, 130, 131
Great Stink, 109
Greenhow, Edward, Dr, 112, 113, 115, 119, 120
Greville, Charles (diarist), 72, 92
Griboyedov, Alexander, 47

Hall, John (Dr), 23, 44, 50, 51, 52, 55, 61, 86, 87, 88, 90, 96, 98, 101, 111, 112, 115, 116, 155, 157
Hardinge, Lord, 62
Harley Street, 16, 19, 20, 74, 140
Herbert, Elizabeth, 11, 16, 130, 131
Herbert, Sidney, 8, 11, 13, 17, 19, 20, 23, 31, 32, 34, 36, 39, 48, 50, 51, 52, 53, 54, 55, 63, 66, 71, 75, 85, 86, 87, 88, 89, 90, 91, 92, 93, 94, 95, 96, 97, 98, 102, 104, 108, 110, 112, 117, 123, 126, 128, 129, 130, 131, 132, 133, 135, 137, 138, 139, 140, 151, 153, 154, 155, 156
Hughes, Amy, 134
Hunt, Mrs (soldier's mother), 29

Inkerman (battle), 24

Joan of Arc, 52

Kaiserswerth, 14
Kinglake, Alexander, 139, 149
Kulali, 50

Lea Hurst, 10, 12, 16, 18, 56
Lefroy, Colonel John, 51, 62, 138, 139, 140, 150, 151
life expectancy, change in, 67, 109, 119, 120, 157
Longfellow, 54
Lucan, 61, 70, 78

Macdonald, Mr. (from *The Times*),24, 33
MacGrigor, Alexander, 33, 34, 35, 36, 39, 42, 43

Malvern, 106, 108
Manning, Cardinal, 13, 138
Martineau, Harriet, 150, 151
masturbation, 15
mathematics, 9, 102
McDonald, Lynn (biographer), 156, 157
McKeown, Thomas, 119, 157
McNeill, Sir John, 38, 39, 40, 41, 42, 43, 44, 45, 46, 47, 48, 49, 50, 51, 52, 55, 57, 58, 59, 60, 61, 62, 63, 64, 65, 66, 69, 70, 71, 73, 74, 80, 82, 83, 84, 88, 94, 96, 98, 102, 103, 130, 132, 137, 138, 140, 141, 142, 148, 155, 156, 157
Menzies, Dr., 23
Mill, John Stuart, 134
Milnes, Richard Monckton, 15, 16, 36
Mouat, James, Dr, 86, 87, 88, 89
Moyser, Mary, 35, 36

Nemesis, 128
Newcastle, Duke of, 20, 75, 102
Nicholas, Tsar, 21
Nightingale Fund, 54, 57, 66, 95, 104, 117, 118, 134
Nightingale Training School, 95, 152
Nightingale, Frances (mother), 7, 8, 9, 13, 14, 15, 17, 31, 36, 54, 55, 56, 102, 103, 105, 108, 152
Nightingale, Parthenope, 7, 9, 14, 29, 53, 81, 102, 103, 106, 152
Nightingale, W. E. (father), 7, 8, 9, 10, 11, 14, 17, 48, 50, 52, 54, 63, 64, 81, 102, 103, 106, 108, 128, 141, 143
Notes on Nursing, 95, 120, 126, 135, 151, 157

O'Malley, Ida (biographer), 13, 14

Palmerston, Lord, 10, 11, 36, 37, 38, 39, 40, 42, 46, 47, 51, 53, 55, 58, 59, 60, 64, 69, 70, 71, 72, 75, 76, 80, 81, 86, 110, 129, 151

Panmure, Lord (Minister of War), 63, 64, 94, 130, 131, 137, 138
Paulet, Lord William, 42, 52
Pennington, Hugh, 157
Persia, 42, 46, 47, 48, 49, 71
potato famine, 46

Quetelet, Adolphe, 18, 102, 143, 144, 147

Raglan, Lord, 31, 43, 45, 50, 85, 87, 90, 99, 100, 106, 123, 143
Rawlinson, Robert, 42, 77, 78, 79, 156
Roberts, Mrs, 48
Royal Commission (1857), 63, 64, 69, 72, 85, 87, 88, 89, 90, 93, 94, 96, 97, 98, 102, 103, 104, 105, 106, 112, 113, 115, 117, 126, 128, 130, 131, 135, 140, 149

Sanitary Commission, 42, 58, 69, 72, 74, 76, 77, 78, 84, 86, 96, 97, 99, 101, 110, 111, 113, 115, 128, 130, 132, 138, 139, 149, 156
'Sanitary', meaning of the word, 89
Scutari, 5, 6, 19, 20, 22, 23, 24, 25, 26, 27, 28, 29, 30, 31, 33, 35, 36, 37, 38, 39, 42, 43, 44, 48, 49, 50, 53, 65, 66, 68, 69, 72, 73, 74, 76, 78, 80, 81, 82, 83, 84, 86, 87, 88, 90, 93, 94, 95, 96, 97, 98, 99, 101, 102, 104, 105, 106, 107, 109, 110, 115, 116, 117, 118, 119, 122, 123, 129, 130, 131, 132, 133, 134, 137, 138, 139, 140, 143, 144, 147, 149, 150, 151, 152, 153, 154, 155, 157
Seacole, Mary, 32, 151
Sebastopol, 22, 24, 25, 37, 46, 47, 55, 130, 135
Shaftesbury, Lord, 74, 76
Shaw Stewart, Jane, 32
Simon, John, 76, 77, 78, 80, 110, 111, 112, 113, 114, 115, 116, 117, 118, 119, 120, 122, 125, 128, 131, 135, 136, 152, 157

Smith, Angus, Dr, 135
Snow, John, Dr, 106, 118, 119
Socinianism, 8
Soyer, Alexis, 135
St Thomas's hospital, 111, 112, 116, 117, 118, 120, 134, 152
Strachey, Lytton, 121, 122, 123
Suggestions for Thought, 18, 141, 142, 143, 144, 145, 147, 149
Sutherland, John, Dr, 42, 58, 69, 74, 76, 77, 78, 79, 84, 96, 99, 106, 110, 111, 115, 116, 121, 131, 132, 133, 135, 138, 140

The Builder, 113, 115, 116
Tulloch, Colonel Alexander, 41, 42, 58, 59, 60, 61, 62, 64, 65, 66, 68, 69, 70, 71, 72, 78, 80, 83, 84, 96, 100, 101, 130, 132, 139, 140, 148, 156
Unitarianism, 7, 8, 9, 13, 18, 52, 125, 144

Victoria, Queen, 21, 39, 40, 41, 46, 47, 53, 54, 59, 60, 62, 63, 64, 70, 88, 138, 152

Wellington, Duke of, 40, 46, 59, 93
Wilson, James, 42
Woodham-Smith, Mrs Cecil (biographer), 124, 152, 154

Young, David, Dr, 123, 124, 125, 154